Public Health: Practices, Methods and Policies

Joav Merrick (Series Editor)
Division for Intellectual and Developmental Disabilities, Ministry of Social Affairs and Social Services, Jerusalem, Israel

"Public Health" is a book series with publications from a multidisciplinary group of researchers, practitioners and clinicians for an international professional forum interested in the broad spectrum of public health issues.

About the Editor-in-Chief
Joav Merrick, MD, MMedSci, DMSc, born and educated in Denmark is Professor of Pediatrics affiliated with the Division of Pediatrics, Hadassah Hebrew University Medical Center, Mt Scopus Campus, Jerusalem, Israel, Kentucky Children's Hospital, University of Kentucky, Lexington, United States and Professor of Public Health at the Center for Healthy Development, School of Public Health, Georgia State University, Atlanta, United States, the former medical director of the Disability Administration, Ministry of Social Affairs and Social Services, Jerusalem and the founder and director of the National Institute of Child Health and Human Development in Israel. Email: jmerrick@zahav.net.il

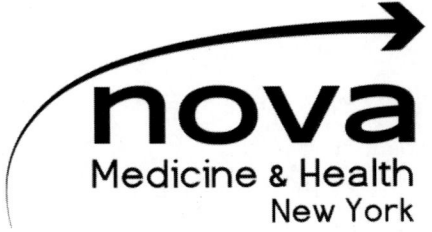

Public Health: Practices, Methods and Policies

Public Health: Implications of Health Behaviors and Diseases
Emmanuel O. Keku, MD, MA, MSPH (Editor)
Joav Merrick, MD, MMedSci, DMSc (Editor)
2023. ISBN: 979-8-89113-083-8 (Hardcover)
2023. ISBN: 979-8-89113-232-0 (eBook)

Positive Youth Development: The Tin Ka Ping P.A.T.H.S. Project in Mainland China
Daniel T.L. Shek, PhD, FHKPS, BBS, SBS, (Editor)
Moon YM Law, RSW, MSW, (Editor)
Xiaoqin Zhu, (Editor)
Joav Merrick, MD, MMedSci, DMSc (Editor)
2022. ISBN: 979-8-88697-282-5 (Softcover)
2022. ISBN: 979-8-88697-324-2 (eBook)

Public Health: Recent International Research
Joav Merrick, MD, MMedSci, DMSc (Editor), Mohammed Morad, MD (Editor)
2022. ISBN: 978-1-68507-491-3 (Hardcover)
2022. ISBN: 978-1-68507-638-2 (eBook)

Environmental Justice and the Intersection of Poverty, Racism and Child Health Disparities
I. Leslie Rubin, MD (Editor), Joav Merrick, MD, MMedSci, DMSc (Editor)
2022. ISBN: 978-1-68507-489-0 (Hardcover)
2022. ISBN: 978-1-68507-640-5 (eBook)

Science, Culture, and Politics: Despair and Hope in the Time of a Pandemic
Consolato M. Sergi, MD (Author)
2021. ISBN: 978-1-53619-816-4 (Hardcover)
2021. ISBN: 978-1-68507-161-5 (eBook)

More information about this series can be found at
https://novapublishers.com/product-category/series/public-health-practices-methods-and-policies/

I. Leslie Rubin
and Joav Merrick
Editors

Environmental Health Disparities

Cultivating Future Leaders

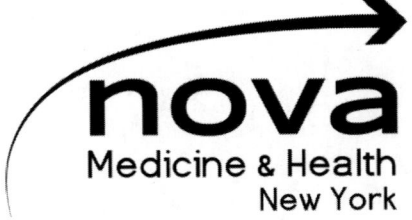

Copyright © 2024 by Nova Science Publishers, Inc.

https://doi.org/10.52305/JWMK4075

All rights reserved. No part of this book may be reproduced, stored in a retrieval system or transmitted in any form or by any means: electronic, electrostatic, magnetic, tape, mechanical photocopying, recording or otherwise without the written permission of the Publisher.

We have partnered with Copyright Clearance Center to make it easy for you to obtain permissions to reuse content from this publication. Please visit copyright.com and search by Title, ISBN, or ISSN.

For further questions about using the service on copyright.com, please contact:

Phone: +1-(978) 750-8400   Copyright Clearance Center   E-mail: info@copyright.com
Fax: +1-(978) 750-4470

NOTICE TO THE READER

The Publisher has taken reasonable care in the preparation of this book but makes no expressed or implied warranty of any kind and assumes no responsibility for any errors or omissions. No liability is assumed for incidental or consequential damages in connection with or arising out of information contained in this book. The Publisher shall not be liable for any special, consequential, or exemplary damages resulting, in whole or in part, from the readers' use of, or reliance upon, this material. Any parts of this book based on government reports are so indicated and copyright is claimed for those parts to the extent applicable to compilations of such works.

Independent verification should be sought for any data, advice or recommendations contained in this book. In addition, no responsibility is assumed by the Publisher for any injury and/or damage to persons or property arising from any methods, products, instructions, ideas or otherwise contained in this publication.

This publication is designed to provide accurate and authoritative information with regards to the subject matter covered herein. It is sold with the clear understanding that the Publisher is not engaged in rendering legal or any other professional services. If legal or any other expert assistance is required, the services of a competent person should be sought. FROM A DECLARATION OF PARTICIPANTS JOINTLY ADOPTED BY A COMMITTEE OF THE AMERICAN BAR ASSOCIATION AND A COMMITTEE OF PUBLISHERS.

Library of Congress Cataloging-in-Publication Data

ISBN: 979-8-89113-487-4

Published by Nova Science Publishers, Inc. † New York

Contents

Introduction 1

Chapter 1   **17th Annual Break the Cycle of children's environmental health disparities program and student projects**..3
I Leslie Rubin, Abby Mutic, Victoria Green, Rebecca Philipsborn, Melissa Gittinger, Jinbing Bai, Nathan Mutic, Wayne Garfinkel, Henry Falk, Benjamin A Gitterman and Joav Merrick

Section one: Break the Cycle 23

Chapter 2   **Break the Cycle program outcomes: Perspectives from a mentor** 25
Jacqueline MacDonald Gibson

Chapter 3   **Break the Cycle: Challenges and impacts in Latin American communities** 37
Patricia M Valenzuela, M Rosario Moore, María Soledad Matus, María I Eugenin, Alejandra Nuñez-Palma and Javiera Martínez-Gutiérrez

Chapter 4   **Factors influencing inequities in lead exposure in United States children: A systematic review**..............51
Michelle Del Rio and Jacqueline MacDonald Gibson

Chapter 5   **Characterizing lead exposure in households that depend on private wells for drinking water** 81
Alyson Alde, Frank Stillo, Abhishek Komandur, James Harrington and Jacqueline MacDonald Gibson

Chapter 6	**The more you know:** **Insights from integrated pre-visit surveys in a** **Pediatric Environmental Health Center** .... 101 Shalini H Shah, Alan D Woolf, Kimberly Manning, Faye Holder-Niles, Bridget Tully, Shelby Flanagan, Matthew C Spence and Marissa Hauptman
Chapter 7	**Increasing maternal education modifies the** **relationship between maternal disorders during** **pregnancy and later life positive child health** **among individuals born extremely preterm** .... 117 Margaret Pinder
Chapter 8	**Factors that influence environmental health** **literacy from returning polycyclic aromatic** **hydrocarbon exposure results** .... 137 Kylie W Riley, Kimberly Burke, Anabel Cole, Maricela Ureno, Holly M Dixon, Lehyla Calero, Lisa M Bramer, Katrina M Waters, Kim A Anderson, Julie B Herbstman and Diana Rohlman

Section two: Acknowledgements 163

About the editors 165

About the Break the Cycle of Health Disparities Inc 167

About the Pediatric Environmental Health Specialty Units
    (PEHSU) 169

About the National Institute of Child Health and Human
    Development in Israel 173

Section three: Index 177

Index 179

Introduction

Chapter 1

17th Annual Break the Cycle of children's environmental health disparities program and student projects

I Leslie Rubin[1-5,*], MD
Abby Mutic[3,6], APRN, PhD
Victoria Green[3,7], JD MD
Rebecca Philipsborn[2,3], MD, MPA
Melissa Gittinger[3,8], DO
Jinbing Bai[3,6], PhD, RN
Nathan Mutic[3,6]
Wayne Garfinkel[3,9], BSCE
Henry Falk[3], MD, MPH
Benjamin A Gitterman[10], MD
and Joav Merrick[11-15], MD, MMedSci, DMSc

[1]Department of Pediatrics, Morehouse School of Medicine, Atlanta, Georgia, United States of America
[2]Department of Pediatrics, Emory University School of Medicine, Atlanta, Georgia, United States of America
[3]Southeast Pediatric Environmental Health Specialty Unit, Emory University, Atlanta, Georgia, United States of America

---

* *Correspondence:* I Leslie Rubin, MD, Associate Professor, Department of Pediatrics, Morehouse School of Medicine, Director, Break the Cycle Program of the Southeast Pediatric Environmental Health Specialty Unit at Emory University, Founder, Break the Cycle of Health Disparities Inc, Medical Director, The Rubin Center for Autism and Developmental Pediatrics. 750 Hammond Drive, Building 1, Suite 100, Atlanta, GA 30342, United States. Email: lrubi01@emory.edu.

In: Environmental Health Disparities
Editors: I. Leslie Rubin and Joav Merrick
ISBN: 979-8-89113-487-4
© 2024 Nova Science Publishers, Inc.

[4]Break the Cycle of Health Disparities Inc, Atlanta, Georgia, United States of America
[5]The Rubin Center for Autism and Developmental Pediatrics, Atlanta, Georgia, United States of America
[6]Nell Hodgson Woodruff School of Nursing, Emory University, Atlanta, Georgia, United States of America
[7]Department of Gynecology and Obstetrics, Emory University School of Medicine, Atlanta, Georgia, United States of America
[8]Georgia Poison Center, Grady Health System, Atlanta, Georgia, United States of America
[9]Retired EPA Region 4 Children's Environmental Health Coordinator, Atlanta, Georgia, United States of America
[10]Departments of Pediatrics and Public Health, George Washington University Schools of Medicine and Public Health and Health Services, General and Community Pediatrics, Children's National Medical Center, Washington DC, United States of America
[11]National Institute of Child Health and Human Development, Jerusalem, Israel
[12]Office of the Medical Director, Health Services, Division for Intellectual and Developmental Disabilities, Ministry of Social Affairs and Social Services, Jerusalem, Israel
[13]Division of Pediatrics, Hadassah Hebrew University Medical Center, Mt Scopus Campus, Jerusalem, Israel
[14]Kentucky Children's Hospital, University of Kentucky College of Medicine, Lexington, Kentucky, United States of America
[15]Center for Human Development, School of Public Health, Georgia State University, Atlanta, Georgia, United States of America

Abstract

The consequences of poverty on the health and well-being of children are clear in the data on health disparities and access to quality healthcare. Income-related disparities are compounded and multiplied by the impact of racial disparities. The human costs in loss of earning potential and the added economic costs to society in supporting such large populations of poor children in poor physical, social, and emotional health, takes its toll on the whole of society. It is incumbent upon all of us to recognize these disparities and inequities in order to develop strategies to reduce the disparities and promote health equity for all children. In this spirit, we offer the *Break the Cycle* program as a model for developing creative strategies while, at the same time, cultivating future leaders to make positive changes to our society. *Break the Cycle* is an annual, collaborative interdisciplinary research and training program involving university students in academic tracks that focus on the impact of adverse social, economic, and environmental factors on children's health, development, and education. Each participating university student develops a project that focuses on preventing or reducing environment-related disorders for children who live in communities where environmental hazards and emotional stresses are related to circumstances of social and economic disadvantage. In this book you will find some of the research projects from the 2021-2022 annual program.

Introduction

While people of all ages are vulnerable to toxic environmental factors that adversely affect their health, children are more vulnerable. Children breathe more air, drink more water, and eat more food for their body weight than adults, so their exposure load through polluted air, water and soil is greater. Furthermore, their organs and organ systems as well as physiologic and metabolic processes are still in the process of development, so they are less likely to metabolize and excrete harmful toxins and therefore are more vulnerable to the toxic effects of the chemicals with immediate and long-term negative health outcomes. For example, children are more vulnerable to air pollution that causes and exacerbates asthma, and to the impact of lead that causes brain damage. Most significantly, children who are exposed to harmful chemicals in early life, even before birth, can have lifelong consequences that affect their health and functional potential, and reduce their opportunities for success in later life (1).

Children who grow up in poverty are most vulnerable to a cumulative set of factors. They are more likely to live in areas where they are exposed to a greater pollution load. Housing in poor neighborhoods tend to be older and therefore more likely to have lead paint (2). Children who live in these older houses are, therefore, more likely to be exposed to lead and have high blood lead levels. Lead causes brain damage in children that results in cognitive impairment, with learning difficulties, attention deficit hyperactivity disorder (ADHD) and behavior problems including aggression (3, 4). The consequent impairment in brain function adversely affects children's ability to learn and achieve success academically, making it less likely that they will graduate from high school and have limited employment opportunities and earning potential. The cumulative impact of these factors on vulnerable children will keep them in low-paying jobs and limit their opportunities for escaping from poverty.

Furthermore, the schools in poor neighborhoods tend to be inadequately funded, because some of the funding support for schools is dependent on property taxes, which in poor communities are obviously low (5). It follows, therefore, that poor neighborhoods have low-income families, which results in lower tax revenue, and consequently low funding for the local school system. Poor funding for schools affects the state of repair of the school buildings and the quality of the indoor environment, as well as the salaries of the teachers and staff and, ultimately, the quality of education for the students (6, 7). The cumulative impact of poverty, lead exposure, and poor education, results in lower academic scores, and a greater likelihood for children to fail grades and drop out of school and thereafter, struggle for gainful employment and a living wage (8, 9).

Children who live in poorer urban neighborhoods are also more likely to live near roadways, where the air is more heavily polluted with exhaust from motor vehicles, increasing the risks for asthma. Also, older houses in these neighborhoods are more likely to have malfunctioning heating and air ventilation systems, resulting in the growth of mold, especially in wetter climates. The presence of mold correlates with a higher likelihood of allergies and asthma and associated adverse consequences on health, including emergency room visits for acute episodes of reactive airway disease with a greater likelihood of absences from school and more hospitalizations with increased mortality (4, 10, 11).

Poor neighborhoods are also more likely to be situated near factories or other sources of pollution of toxic waste, which may result in poor air quality and poor water and soil quality. These conditions, taken together, impact children in poverty and their families disproportionately and cumulatively (8). The placement of factories and polluting industries near poor neighborhoods puts affected communities at risk for a variety of adverse health outcomes related to the pollution and constitutes an environmental injustice (12, 13).

Thus, children who grow up in poverty are more likely to be exposed to multiple adverse physical, chemical, and social elements in their environment and are more likely to be emotionally stressed, with feelings of insecurity, anxiety and fear (14). The combination of emotional and environmental stresses takes a toll on the physiological, neurological, immunological, educational, and psychological well-being of children. These cumulative stressors have metabolic and hemodynamic consequences on their cardiovascular, immune, and endocrine systems, resulting in an increased likelihood of adverse health outcomes in adulthood, such as obesity, diabetes, and hypertension (15).

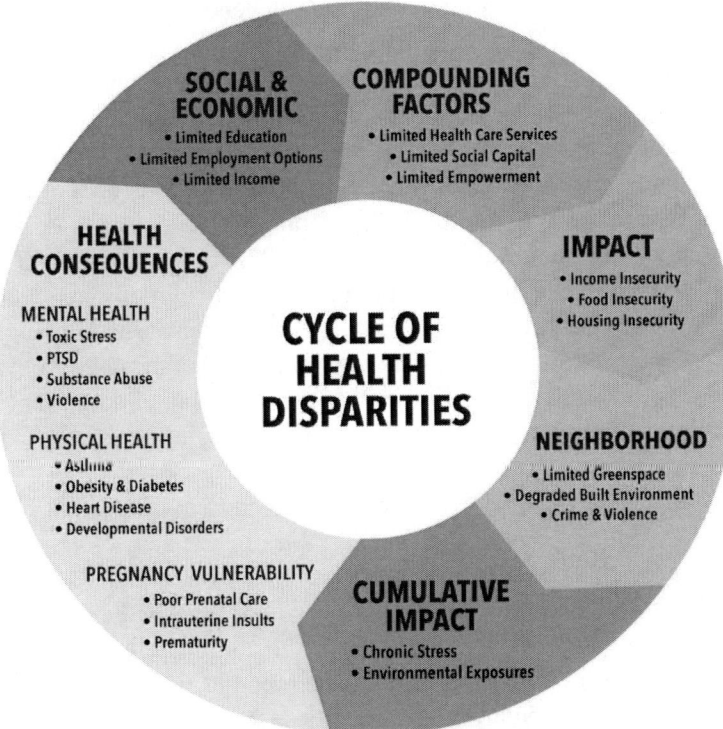

Figure 1. Cycle of environmental health disparities (24).

Furthermore, the neighborhood environment in poor areas, with crowded houses, greater likelihood of vehicular traffic, poor lighting, and likely presence of trash, provide the dystopian setting for a drug culture, crime, and violence, with little to no green spaces and suitable facilities for safe and healthy recreation (4, 16). These conditions increase the risks for crime with fear of assault, and a greater likelihood of being children being exposed to street drugs and drug dealers, with an increased likelihood of gun violence (17).

As children reach adolescence, they are more likely to experience school failure and engage in risky behaviors, such as substance abuse, gang membership, and contribute to the prevalence of crime and violence. Many of these young people drop out of school and face limited employment options, and they are more likely to carry a relatively dim view of their future, resort to drugs to feel better or crime to make money to survive or support their habits and lifestyles. These behaviors can result in incarceration, or in the most extreme instances, death from drugs or gun violence, with the emotional and social consequences for the individual, the family, the community and society (18, 19). This scenario plays out in too many cities in the United States (US), which has the highest incarceration rate in the world with a disproportionate percentage of young men of color in prison (20). It is noteworthy and reason for a modicum of optimism that, since its peak in the 1990s with over 100,000 children in prison, the number of juvenile justice cases has decreased substantially, but remains at a disturbing 36,000 with more than 500 children under 12 years of age in in prison in 2019 (21). Although this positive trend is a result of local, state, and federal processes, making positive change in the lives of vulnerable children, it begins with taking individual action and striving to make a positive difference in the lives of vulnerable children; not only in reducing the negative environmental factors, but in promoting resilience through education as well as emotional and social support (22).

The assault of adverse social, economic, and environmental factors on vulnerable children results in unfavorable health, developmental, and educational outcomes and compromises a child's opportunity for economic and social success in life (23). This persistent pattern devolves into the perpetuation of an intergenerational cycle, the codification of which, can be represented in an ecological construct that embodies the concept of the cycle of children's environmental health disparities (see Figure 1) (24).

Intersection of poverty, race/ethnicity, and child health in the United States

There is a significant difference in race and ethnicity among poor children. The Children's Defense Fund reports that approximately 1 in 3 African American children, 1 in 3 Native American children and nearly 1 in 4 Hispanic American children were living in poverty compared with 1 in 11 White children, and that almost two-thirds of Black, Hispanic, and Native American children live in areas of concentrated poverty, compared with one-third of White children (25). This disparity in poverty correlates with a disparity in infant mortality rate in the US, which is more than double in the Black (10.8) and almost double in Native American (8.2) populations compared to the White population (4.6) (26).

The centuries-long history of slavery and continued political and economic oppression and suppression of people of color, whether they be of

African descent, Indigenous descent, or from other parts of the world such as Latin America, has resulted in the concentration of poverty in communities of color across the US (27). There are clear political and economic factors that continue to play a significant role in creating the disproportionate environmental impacts on the affected individuals, communities, and populations (27). Discrimination and bias leveled at groups of people is racism and expresses itself at many levels of society, from the individual interaction, through provision of services, such as healthcare and education, to employment, career advancement, social status, and all manner of social and economic life (28). Racism exacerbates and aggravates the impact of poverty on children's health disparities. This phenomenon has led the CDC to declare that racism *negatively affects the mental and physical health of millions of people, preventing them from attaining their highest level of health, and consequently, affecting the health of our nation* (29). The American Academy of Pediatrics identifies racism as a core social determinant of health linked to birth disparities, adverse physical and mental health problems in children and adolescents, and ongoing health problems that manifest in adulthood, thus reducing life expectancy and adding costs to society (30).

Break the Cycle program

Break the Cycle is an annual, collaborative interdisciplinary research and training program involving university students in academic tracks that focus on the impact of adverse social, economic, and environmental factors on children's health, development, and education. Each participating university student develops a project that focuses on preventing or reducing environment-related disorders for children who live in communities where environmental hazards and emotional stresses are related to circumstances of social and economic disadvantage. At the conclusion of the project period, the students present the results of their projects at a national conference and write manuscripts on their projects for publication in a peer-reviewed journal supplement dedicated to the collection of projects from each annual program.

The annual program begins with a call for proposals from a wide range of university students. Proposals are evaluated by a competitive review process for the quality of the proposal, its relevance to children's environmental health disparities, creativity, and feasibility. Each year the top students are selected to work with their academic mentors and their home universities, and with *Break the Cycle* faculty, to complete their projects. The students and their mentors are required to participate in monthly conference calls, during which the progress of each project is reviewed, additional perspectives are explored, and constructive guidance is provided. During these conference calls, students and their mentors also have an opportunity to communicate and collaborate with their counterparts at other universities.

Fundamental to *Break the Cycle* is the expectation that the projects make a positive difference by improving the health and well-being of children, their families, and their communities. It is also envisioned that the students would be inspired to pursue careers that focus on reducing health disparities and in becoming leaders for the future. Furthermore, because each student is required to have a mentor at their home university, it is anticipated that the faculty mentors add to the literature and body of science on the subject into their curricula, and thereby promote further research and academic interest in this field (see Table 1).

Table 1. Project guidelines

- University faculty identify students who have an interest in this topic area and support the student in the selection of an idea for projects that explore environmental factors that adversely affect the health of children living in circumstances of social and economic disadvantage. Alternatively, students interested in a specific project can initiate the application process and identify mentors to work with them.
- The students submit their proposals which are reviewed by the *Break the Cycle* faculty. The process is competitive with only 10 projects being selected each year.
- During the project period, there are monthly conference calls with all students and mentors to monitor the progress of their projects, share ideas, and assure that the projects are consistent with the spirit of the *Break the Cycle* concept.
- At the end of the project period, the students present the results of their work at the annual *Break the Cycle* conference.
- The students are then required to write papers on their projects, which are submitted for publication in an international journal as a monograph of the *Break the Cycle* projects. The papers are also published as chapters in a book as part of a public health series.
- The progress and careers of the participating students are tracked to evaluate the impact of their participation in the *Break the Cycle* program

Table 2. Desired outcomes

• To inspire students from a variety of academic disciplines to explore the impact of adverse social, economic, environmental, and political factors on the health, development, and education of children, and to creatively generate strategies to address the challenges.
• To collaborate with an interdisciplinary team of academic leaders from a variety of different universities and colleges to get a perspective on the broader issues of this topic area.
• To encourage faculty at universities who participate in this program to promote academic interest and social awareness in children's environmental health disparities.
• To cultivate future leaders among the students.

It is also anticipated that participating students inspire peers in their academic, professional, and social circles, and that the interdisciplinary nature of the program with participation of students at other universities around the world be stimulating and inspiring (see Table 2). A 2012 survey of alumni of the program demonstrates that students derive significant benefit from all aspects of their participation in the process, which include the practical aspects of conducting a research project, in preparing and delivering a presentation, and in writing a manuscript. The manuscripts, which are published in this volume, provide the students with an asset for further academic or employment opportunities. Each student gains knowledge about children's environmental health and environmental health disparities as well as being exposed to different perspectives from the other student projects. Many participants report that their participation in the program influenced their career choice (31).

Since its inception in 2004, *Break the Cycle* has held 17 annual programs and worked with over 150 students representing 50 different university departments in 12 states in the US, as well as students from countries in Latin America, Europe, and Africa. To date, 13 monographs have been published in international journals and 13 books in a public health series. In the 2012 survey, alumni rated their experience with *Break the Cycle* as valuable, with many reporting that they pursued careers relating to their *Break the Cycle* projects (31).

Commentaries from mentors on Break the Cycle

Mentors from the universities and colleges have played a significant role in recruiting and supporting the trainees with their projects, their presentations and their publications, as well as contributing to our collective learning experiences. More than that, they have played a key role in helping achieve our Desired Outcomes (see Table 2). When we articulated the outcome: *To encourage faculty at universities who participate in this program to promote academic interest and social awareness in children's environmental health disparities,* what we did not realize was the extent to which the mentors embraced the concepts and spirit of the *Break the Cycle* program, and how it helped shape some of their work. In this volume we include 2 contributions from mentors who have participated over multiple years with multiple students.

Break the Cycle program outcomes: Perspectives from a mentor

Jacqueline MacDonald Gibson, PhD: Department of Civil, Construction, and Environmental Engineering, North Carolina State University Raleigh, North Carolina, United States of America.

I have participated in six years of Break the Cycle (BTC) projects with mentees who helped to decrease disparities in exposure to lead (Pb) in drinking water in North Carolina. These mentees' projects documented that inequitable access to a regulated community water supply in African American neighborhoods bordering some North Carolina cities and towns exposes children to elevated water lead (Pb). One BTC mentee found elevated water Pb in 28% of homes in affected areas—a prevalence similar to that in Flint, Michigan, during the water crisis. In a large epidemiologic study (n = 34,314), another mentee revealed that living in areas without municipal water service was associated with a highly significant increase $(p < 0.001)$ in children's blood Pb. A third mentee measured Pb in water, blood, and dust in 75 households without community water, finding that water filters significantly decreased Pb in water and, consequently, in blood. However, there were significant racial disparities in access to filters: 38% of African and Native Americans had a filter, compared to 83% of participants of other races. A fourth mentee constructed a socioecological model showing that high Pb in water in these communities' compounds risks among a population demographic group (African Americans) that also is disproportionately exposed to Pb from other environmental sources. Data collected through these projects helped one community win its battle for community water service, resulting in a 70% decrease in Pb in drinking water. The projects inspired mentees to pursue additional graduate training and careers in environmental health research and consulting.

Break the Cycle: Challenges and impacts in Latin American communities

Patricia M Valenzuela, MD, MSc: Department of Pediatrics, Facultad de Medicina, Pontificia Universidad Católica de Chile, Santiago, Chile.

The Break the Cycle (BTC) program was developed to promote quality research focusing on underserved communities, for example, covering prevalent issues that affect underserved communities in Latin America. Three Chilean studies were developed with BTC support. The students were pediatric residents whose research topics were discussed with their Chilean mentors and the BTC team. The main results of these studies were the following: 1) Identification of increased awareness of indoor environmental risk factors for pediatric respiratory diseases in an underserved community: 50 families, 32% of children had past illnesses (87.5% asthma); 24% reported smoking happening in the home; 62% had animals living indoors. 2) Screening for autism; Community perspectives: We screened 200 children (16 to 30 months of age) with the M-CHAT and M-CHAT follow-up interview (MC-FUI) in middle-low and very low socioeconomic and vulnerable communities: 22% screened positive; 11.4% of them continued to be at risk after the MC-FUI; and two children were confirmed for ASD. 3) Measuring parenting dimensions and social and prosocial abilities in adolescents living in vulnerable families. 120 adolescents reported that most caregivers had an authoritative parenting style. There was a correlation between high parenting demandingness and monitoring, with high prosocial skills among adolescents. Conclusions: The BTC program created great opportunities for students and mentors to improve and expand their research by including the social determinants of health. Being more aware of social disparities helped them to focus on finding ways to break the cycle.

Break the Cycle 17 projects

The papers in this publication represent the interdisciplinary array of creative work by students from universities in the United States who participated in the 17th Annual *Break the Cycle* program in 2022. As usual, the papers in this volume cover a wide range of topic areas, including the critical importance of exposure to toxic chemicals, particularly lead, the importance of clean air and clean water, social determinants of birth outcomes, health literacy and environmental health literacy, and the role of pediatric environmental health clinics.

Factors influencing inequities in lead exposure in United States children: A systematic review

Student: Michelle Del Rio MPH, PhD
Mentor: Jaqueline MacDonald Gibson PhD
Department of Environmental and Occupational Health, Indiana University Bloomington, Bloomington, Indiana and Department of Civil, Construction, and Environmental Engineering, North Carolina State University, Raleigh, North Carolina, United States of America

Abstract

Although US policies to limit lead (Pb) release into the environment have substantially decreased children's blood Pb concentrations over the past four decades, more than a million children are still exposed to harmful Pb levels. A social-ecological model (SEM) of childhood Pb exposure may help public health professionals and government officials prevent these exposures by identifying the combinations of individual and social environmental factors that have resisted previous Pb exposure control policies and programs. To develop such an SEM, we conducted a systematic review of studies of children's blood Pb in the United States published since 2005. Information on risk factors for Pb exposure was extracted from each article. Identified risk factors were then grouped into the five levels of an SEM: intrapersonal, interpersonal, institutional, community, and public policy. In total, the review identified 75 peer-reviewed studies of children's Pb exposure in the United States. The review revealed that while child blood Pb levels have declined over time, inequities of Pb exposure persist among Non-Hispanic Black, migrant, and low-income children. Mixed effects were reported for Hispanic/Latinx/Mexican-American populations, with some studies finding these groups were at higher risk and others showing lower risks. Surprisingly, some studies found higher blood Pb in children over age 5 than in younger children, though the reverse was generally true. Findings reveal new opportunities to target exposure prevention programs at the intrapersonal, institutional, community, and policy levels. Well-controlled studies of the effectiveness of interventions at each level are needed to guide future policymaking.

Characterizing lead exposure in households that depend on private wells for drinking water

Student: Alyson Alde MS
Mentor: Jacqueline MacDonald Gibson PhD
Department of Environmental and Occupational Health,
School of Public Health, Indiana University, Bloomington, Indiana,
Department of Civil, Construction, and Environmental Engineering,
North Carolina State University, Raleigh, North Carolina,
United States of America

Abstract

Evidence accumulated over the past several decades indicates that there is no safe level of exposure to lead. Although the Safe Drinking Water Act limits exposure to lead from municipal water supplies, no such protection exists for private wells. Research suggests United States children relying on private wells have increased risk from lead exposure compared to those served by a regulated water system. However, no prior US studies have concurrently measured water and blood lead levels in homes using private wells. To assess these associations, we collected blood, tap water and household dust samples from 89 participants using private wells for drinking water. A multivariable regression was performed to examine the association between well water lead and blood lead, controlling for lead in dust and other confounders. Although water and blood lead levels were not directly associated, filtering water was associated with a 32% decrease in blood lead ($p < 0.05$). Additionally, using a filter was significantly associated with decreased risk high lead in water ($p = 0.01$). We found significant racial disparities in access to water filters. Among African American or Native American participants, 38% had a water filter, compared to 83% of other participants ($p < 0.001$). This study highlights that drinking unfiltered private well water may increase the risk of exposure to lead and that racial disparities in access to and use of water filters in homes relying on private wells, may therefore contribute to longstanding disparities in children's blood lead.

The more you know: Insights from integrated pre-visit surveys in a pediatric environmental health center

Student: Shalini H Shah DO
Mentor: Marissa Hauptman MD, MPH
Pediatric Environmental Health Center, Boston Children's Hospital, Boston, Massachusetts, Harvard Medical School, Boston, Massachusetts, United States of America

Abstract

The Pediatric Environmental Health Center (PEHC) at Boston Children's Hospital is a specialty referral clinic that provides consultation for approximately 250 patients annually. Identifying environmental hazards is key for clinical management. Exposure concerns include lead, mold, pesticides, perfluoroalkyl substances (PFAS), impaired air quality, and more. Our goal was to identify concerns and visit priorities of our patient population to guide visits. A 47-question pre-visit survey was created exploring potential environmental hazards and administered prior to visits using a platform integrated into the electronic medical record (EMR). The study group was a convenience sample of patients from June 2021 to June 2022. Of 204 total visits, 101 surveys were submitted, yielding a response rate of 49.5%. 66/101 (65.3%) were surveys from initial consultations used for descriptive analysis. The majority of patients were seen for a chief complaint of lead exposure (90.1%). Most respondents had concerns about peeling paint (40.0%), and those reporting peeling paint were more likely to report additional concerns [75.0%, $p < 0.001$]. Other concerns highlighted were mold (15.2%), pests (15.2%), asbestos (10.6%), air pollution (9.1%), temperature regulation (7.6%), pesticides (6.1%), PFAS (4.5%), and formaldehyde (4.5%). A knowledge gap was identified; 45.5% (30/66) respondents responded "no" to the question asking if the Poison Control Center phone number was stored in their phone. This study illustrates how the implementation of a pre-visit EMR integrated survey engages families, informs clinical care, and serves as a point-of-care education tool for specific knowledge gaps. Findings will guide development of future environmental health screeners.

Increasing maternal education modifies the relationship between maternal disorders during pregnancy and later life positive child health among individuals born extremely preterm

Student: Margaret Pinder
Mentor: Rebecca C. Fry
University of North Carolina at Chapel Hill, Gillings School of Global Public Health, Department of Environmental Health Sciences, Chapel Hill, North Carolina, The Institute for Environmental Health Solutions, Gillings School of Global Public Health, The University of North Carolina at Chapel Hill, Chapel Hill, North Carolina, United States of America

Abstract

The extremely low gestational age newborn (ELGAN) study collected data from over 1,506 infants from fourteen hospitals born at 28 weeks' gestation or earlier. At the time of birth, data were collected about maternal health conditions, including pre-pregnancy diabetes, obesity, hypertension and asthma. Follow-up studies were conducted when these individuals were two, ten, and fifteen years old and among the data collected were social and environmental variables, including maternal education. A positive child health index (PCHI) has been developed in order to evaluate adverse health outcomes in later life for ELGANs and to identify antecedents of positive health in childhood. This index was calculated at both the 10-year and 15-year follow-up interviews, and it is known that maternal health conditions at birth can influence PCHI among ELGANs at age 10. The aim of this project was to determine if changes in maternal education between birth and age 15 years moderate the relationship between maternal health conditions and positive child health at age 15 years.

Factors influence environmental health literacy from returning polycyclic aromatic hydrocarbon exposure results

Student: Kylie W Riley, MPH
Mentor: Julie B Herbstman, PhD, MSc
Columbia Center for Children's Environmental Health, Columbia University, New York, United States of America
[2]*Department of Environmental Health Sciences,*
Mailman School of Public Health, Columbia University, New York, United States of America

Abstract

Reporting personal environmental exposure data back from researchers to study participants is becoming more common, however there are few tools to assess whether report back increases environmental health literacy (EHL). This study assessed whether sociodemographic or environmental characteristics were associated with changes in EHL after receiving personal air monitoring results. This study was conducted in a New York City based pregnancy cohort wherein participants were assessed for exposure to polycyclic aromatic hydrocarbons during the third trimester of pregnancy. Participants (n = 168) received their results two to five years after participation and a subset (n = 47) completed a survey evaluating perspectives on their results and subsequent behaviors. Using these results, we created a quantitative scale of EHL, with higher scores indicative of higher EHL. We found that participants with a college degree were significantly more likely to be surprised by their results than those with less than a high school degree (OR = 5.60, $p \leq 0.05$) and that higher naphthalene levels were associated with decreased odds of being surprised about receiving the results (OR = 0.37, $p = 0.02$). There were no observed associations between demographic or exposure characteristics and our dichotomous EHL indicator; however, those with more education and higher income tended to have higher EHL scores. Additionally, participants who reported being surprised by or glad to receive their results had higher EHL scores. Open-ended text responses indicated that while some participants felt worried after receiving their results, participants reported being glad to have received the report.

Conclusion

The consequences of poverty on the health and well-being of children are clear in the data on health disparities and access to quality healthcare. Income-related disparities are compounded and multiplied by the impact of racial disparities. The human costs in loss of earning potential and the added economic costs to society in supporting such large populations of poor children in poor physical, social, and emotional health, takes its toll on the whole of society. It is incumbent upon all of us to recognize these disparities and inequities and develop strategies to reduce the disparities and promote health equity among all children. In this spirit, we offer the *Break the Cycle* program as a model for developing creative strategies while, at the same time, cultivating future leaders to make positive changes to our society.

As a core principle, *Break the Cycle* promotes awareness of the social, economic, and environmental determinants of health and encourages the development of creative and innovative strategies to reduce and eliminate health disparities in our society, for the good of all. As in previous *Break the Cycle* programs, current students benefited from the process of creatively developing a project, translating it into action, performing the research, presenting the results of their projects at a national conference, and writing manuscripts for publication in this journal. Each student project highlights ways to *Break the Cycle* of Children's Environmental Health Disparities through different components of the *Break the Cycle* diagram (see Figure 1):

- To reduce the likelihood of exposure to adverse environmental factors for vulnerable children.
- To improve their environmental circumstances by providing enhanced support, quality education and quality health care.
- To reduce added stressors.
- To promote resilience.

In this process, the students gain valuable knowledge and skills towards becoming the next generation of leaders and building on their knowledge and experience to further the goals of reducing children's environmental health disparities and promoting health equity for all children. This research and training model is a relatively inexpensive and cost-effective way of inspiring young bright students to focus their potential on changing the world for the better by developing research and communication skills and by embodying the principles of justice, equity, and collaboration. In the process, we all gain additional knowledge, understanding and perspective to become more inclusive and open to innovations and progress.

Acknowledgments

Thanks to the additional editors of some of the papers who have given of their time and expertise, much appreciated especially our trusted friend and star guest editor, editor David Ervin, as well as Erin Lebow-Skelly at the HERCULES Project at Emory University Rollins School of Public Health. This publication was supported by the cooperative agreement award number 5 NU61TS000237-05 from the Agency for Toxic Substances and Disease

Registry (ATSDR). Its contents are the responsibility of the authors and do not necessarily represent the official views of the Agency for Toxic Substances and Disease Registry (ATSDR). The US Environmental Protection Agency (EPA) supports the PEHSU by providing partial funding to ATSDR under Inter-Agency Agreement number DW-75-95877701. Neither EPA nor ATSDR endorse the purchase of any commercial products or services mentioned in PEHSU publications.

References

[1] Etzel RA, Balk SJ, eds. Children's unique vulnerabilities to environmental hazards. In: Etzel RA, Balk SJ, eds. Pediatric environmental Health, 4th Edition: Itasca, IL: American Academy of Pediatrics, 2019:17-31.

[2] Kim DY, Staley F, Curtis G, Buchanan S. Relation between housing age, housing value, and childhood blood lead levels in children in Jefferson County, KY. Am J Public Health 2002;92(5):769-72.

[3] Egan KB, Cornwell CR, Courtney JG, Ettinger AS. Blood lead levels in US children ages 1–11 years, 1976–2016. Environ Health Perspect 2021;129(3). doi.org/10.1289/EHP7932.

[4] Adamkiewicz G, Zota AR, Fabian MP, Chahine T, Julien R, Spengler JD, Levy JI. Moving environmental justice indoors: understanding structural influences on residential exposure patterns in low-income communities. Am J Public Health 2011;101(Suppl 1):S238–45.

[5] How do school funding formulas work? URL: https://apps.urban.org/features/funding-formulas/.

[6] Barshay, J. The Hechinger Report: A decade of research on the rich-poor divide in education. URL: https://hechingerreport.org/a-decade-of-research-on-the-rich-poor-divide-in-education/.

[7] Semuels A. Good school, rich school; bad school, poor school: The inequality at the heart of America's education system. The Atlantic 2016 Aug 25. URL: https://www.theatlantic.com/business/archive/2016/08/property-taxes-and-unequal-schools/497333/.

[8] Solomon GM, Morello-Frosch R, Zeise L, Faust JB. Cumulative environmental impacts: Science and policy to protect communities. Annu Rev Public Health 2016;37:83–96.

[9] Faust JB. Perspectives on cumulative risks and impacts. Int J Toxicol 2010;29(1):58-64.

[10] Pacheco CM, Ciaccio CE, Nazir M, Daley CM, DiDonna A,4 Won S. Choi, Barnes CS, P Rosenwasser LJ. Homes of low-income minority families with asthmatic children have increased condition issues. Allergy Asthma Proc 2014;35(6):467–74.

[11] Healthy People 2020. URL: https://www.healthypeople.gov/2020/topics-objectives/topic/social-determinants-health/interventions-resources/quality-of-housing.

[12] National Environmental Justice Advisory Council. Cumulative Risks/Impacts Work Group. Ensuring risk reduction in communities with multiple stressors: Environmental justice and cumulative risks/impacts, 2004. URL: https://www.epa.gov/sites/production/files/2015-04/documents/ensuringriskreducationnejac.pdf.

[13] Pair QC, Environmental justice and the future of America. Int Public Health J 2021;13(4):377-88.

[14] Hodgkinson S, Godoy L, Beers LS. Improving mental health access for low-income children and families in the primary care setting. Pediatrics 2017;139(1):e20151175.

[15] Shonkoff JP, Garner AS, Committee on Psychosocial Aspects of Child and Family Health, Committee on Early Childhood, Adoption, and Dependent Care, Section on Developmental and Behavioral Pediatrics. The lifelong effects of early childhood adversity and toxic stress. Pediatrics 2012;129(1):e232-46.

[16] Hood E. Dwelling disparities: How poor housing leads to poor health. Environ Health Perspect 2005;113(5):A310–7.

[17] Friedman J, Karandinos G, Hart LK, Castrillo FM, Graetz N. Structural vulnerability to narcotics-driven firearm violence: An ethnographic and epidemiological study of Philadelphia's Puerto Rican inner-city. PLoS One 2019;14(11):e0225376.

[18] Rubin IL, Geller RJ, Martinuzzi K, Howett M, Gitterman BA, Wells LM, et al. Children's environmental health disparities: The costs and benefits of breaking the cycle. Int J Child Health Hum Dev 2016;9(4):419-30.

[19] Wodtke GT, Elwert F, Harding DJ. Poor families, poor neighborhoods: How family poverty intensifies the impact of concentrated disadvantage on high school graduation. Ann Arbor, MI: University Michigan, Population Studies Center Research Report 12-776, 2012.

[20] The Sentencing Project. Criminal Justice facts. URL: https://www.sentencingproject.org/criminal-justice-facts/.

[21] Sickmund M, Sladky TJ, Puzzanchera C, Kang W. Easy access to the Census of Juveniles in Residential Placement, 2021. URL: https://www.ojjdp.gov/ojstatbb/ezacjrp/.

[22] Rubin IL. Resilience: A commentary on breaking the cycle. Int Public Health J 2018;10(3):247-64.

[23] Mood C, Jonsson JO. The social consequences of poverty: An empirical test on longitudinal data. Soc Indic Res 2016;127:633–52.

[24] Rubin IL, Geller RJ, Martinuzzi K, Howett M, Gitterman BA, Wells L, et al. Break the cycle of children's environmental health disparities: An ecological framework. Int Public Health J 2017;9(2):115-249.

[25] Children's Defense Fund. State of American Children. URL: https://www.childrensdefense.org/wp-content/uploads/2020/02/The-State-Of-Americas-Children-2020.pdf.

[26] CDC. Infant mortality. URL: https://www.cdc.gov/reproductivehealth/maternalinfanthealth/infantmortality.htm.

[27] Lee C. Confronting disproportionate impacts and systemic racism in environmental policy. Environ Law Reporter 2021 March 10.

[28] Johnson TJ. Intersection of bias, structural racism, and social determinants with health care inequities. Pediatrics 2020;146(2):e2020003657.
[29] CDC. Racism and health. URL: https://www.cdc.gov/minorityhealth/racism-disparities/index.html.
[30] Trent M, Dooley DG, Dougé J. The impact of racism on child and adolescent health. Pediatrics 2019;144(2):e20191765.
[31] Rubin IL, Oves D, Nodvin J, Geller RJ, Howett M, Martinuzzi K, et al. The learning experience of 'Break the Cycle' program: Survey of past students. In: Rubin IL, Merrick J, eds. Environmental health disparities. New York: Nova Science, 2016:171-85.

Section one: Break the Cycle

Chapter 2

Break the Cycle program outcomes: Perspectives from a mentor

Jacqueline MacDonald Gibson[*], PhD
Department of Civil, Construction, and Environmental Engineering,
North Carolina State University Raleigh, North Carolina, United States of America

Abstract

> I have participated in six years of Break the Cycle (BTC) projects with mentees who helped to decrease disparities in exposure to lead (Pb) in drinking water in North Carolina. These mentees' projects documented that inequitable access to a regulated community water supply in African American neighborhoods bordering some North Carolina cities and towns exposes children to elevated water lead (Pb). One BTC mentee found elevated water Pb in 28% of homes in affected areas—a prevalence similar to that in Flint, Michigan, during the water crisis. In a large epidemiologic study (n = 34,314), another mentee revealed that living in areas without municipal water service was associated with a highly significant increase *(p < 0.001)* in children's blood Pb. A third mentee measured Pb in water, blood, and dust in 75 households without community water, finding that water filters significantly decreased Pb in water and, consequently, in blood. However, there were significant racial disparities in access to filters: 38% of African and Native Americans had a filter, compared to 83% of participants of other races. A fourth mentee constructed a socioecological model showing that high Pb in water in these communities compounds risks among a population demographic group (African Americans) that also is disproportionately exposed to Pb

---

[*] ***Correspondence:*** Jacqueline MacDonald Gibson, PhD, Head, Department of Civil, Construction, and Environmental Engineering, North Carolina State University, Raleigh, North Carolina, United States. Email: jmacdon@ncsu.edu.

In: Environmental Health Disparities
Editors: I. Leslie Rubin and Joav Merrick
ISBN: 979-8-89113-487-4
© 2024 Nova Science Publishers, Inc.

from other environmental sources. Data collected through these projects helped one community win its battle for community water service, resulting in a 70% decrease in Pb in drinking water. The projects inspired mentees to pursue additional graduate training and careers in environmental health research and consulting.

Introduction

My students and I began participating in the Break the Cycle (BTC) programs during the 2016–2017 cohort. We wanted to build our skills in applied research to identify and decrease the environment's contribution to health disparities. The BTC program provided an ideal venue to connect with and receive mentoring from scholars with similar interests. My students and I have participated in three BTC cohorts. The common focus in our projects across cohorts has been documenting health disparities arising from inequitable access to safe, reliable access to drinking water in North Carolina (NC). Three students and one post-doctoral mentee have completed the BTC program. Their BTC experiences helped to inform their subsequent education and career choices. Perhaps more importantly, the data they gathered helped one historically African American community resolve its longstanding problems with access to a sufficient supply of safe drinking water.

Setting for BTC projects

My students' BTC projects focused on access to safe drinking water in African American communities located in "extraterritorial jurisdictions" (ETJs) of North Carolina (NC) cities and towns. An ETJ is an area outside of municipal corporate limits that is subject to the municipality's zoning and development regulations. Many states, including NC, allow cities and towns to designate land beyond their borders as part of their ETJ (1). The municipality regulates land use in ETJs, but ETJ residents cannot vote in municipal elections. In addition, they are not guaranteed access to municipal services, including water and wastewater service, trash collection, and municipal fire and police protection. States began allowing municipalities to extend their authority into ETJs more than 100 years ago; in NC, ETJs may extend up to three miles from the municipal boundary. The rationale for granting municipalities this power includes the need to protect public health of municipal residents, since pollution does not respect administrative boundaries (1). However, limited case studies available when we began our BTC research suggested that there may be racial disparities in the quality of water and sanitation services in these areas, but these disparities and the resulting health effects had not been studied systematically (2). Figure 1 shows ETJs across North Carolina.

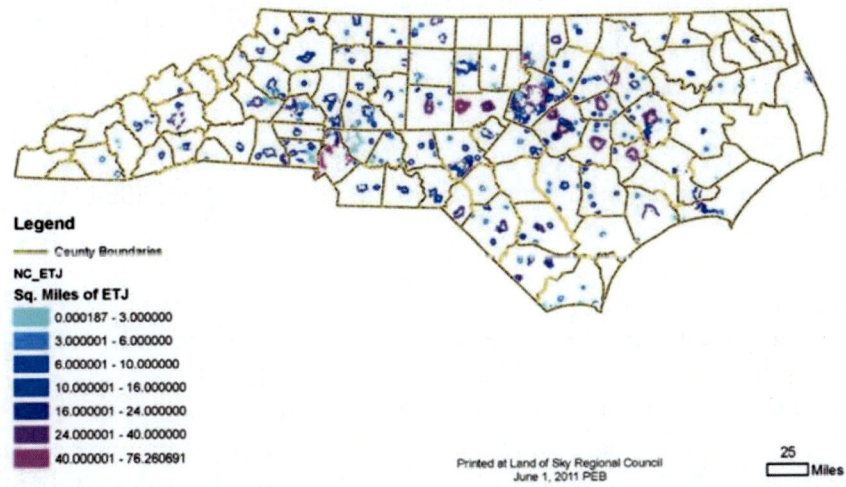

Figure 1. Extraterritorial jurisdictions (ETJs) of municipalities in North Carolina. Associated municipalities are the white-colored areas circled by the ETJs, which are in color.

Although some cities may extend municipal services into ETJs (usually at an increased cost compared to what municipal residents pay), they are not required to do so. When these services are unavailable, ETJ residents must provide for their own water and sanitation needs, typically by drilling their own water wells and installing septic systems. These communities therefore are not afforded the benefits of professional monitoring and management of their water and wastewater systems that are available to municipal residents receiving community services. Instead, when problems arise, ETJ homeowners must manage repairs on their own. Problems may include contamination of the water supply, overflowing septic systems, and unreliable water flow. Climate change may exacerbate these problems due to increases in the frequency of severe storms that may flood and contaminate private wells and inundate septic systems (3). Conversely, climate change may increase the frequency of droughts, leading to an increased frequency of wells running dry (4). My students and I have explored three questions:

1. To what extent is community water service available in NC ETJs, and does service availability vary with the community's racial composition?
2. What is the quality of self-supplied drinking water in ETJs?
3. What are the health consequences (if any) of exclusion from municipal water service in ETJs?

My students' BTC projects have addressed the last two questions. To contextualize their work, I also summarize my findings regarding the first question.

Racial disparities in community water service access in ETJs

Formative research conducted before my first students enrolled in the BTC program identified significant racial disparities in community water service access in NC ETJs. In Wake County, the state's second-largest by population (housing 10% of the NC population), every 10% increase in the African American population proportion of an ETJ census block was associated with a 3.8% decrease in the odds of having community water service, controlling for property value and population density (5). Across NC's 75 rural counties, census blocks that were less than 22% Black had 42% higher odds of having water service than those that were 50-99% Black, and 85% higher odds of water service than 100% Black census blocks, controlling for population density and median home value (6). As the White population proportion in the adjacent municipality increased, the odds that water service would be extended to the corresponding African American ETJ areas decreased significantly. This pattern of excluding communities of color from nearby municipal services has been observed by demographers, who have termed this phenomenon "municipal underbounding" (7–9).

BTC 2016–2017: Water quality in private wells in ETJs

My first mentee to enroll in BTC was Frank Stillo, then a PhD student. His participation in the 2016–2017 cohort catalyzed a project to document the chemical quality of the tap water in ETJ areas excluded from community water service. At the time, the Flint, Michigan, water crisis was in the news, raising national concern about exposure to lead (Pb) in drinking water. (During the crisis, the municipal water system's corrosion control program failed, causing Pb from the water distribution system and household plumbing to leach into the tap water of the city's residents.) We found that only one small study had investigated the occurrence of Pb in drinking water in an ETJ community (10). The study found high Pb levels in one of 12 wells tested; a major limitation was that the sampling protocol relied on a "flushed" water sample collected after the kitchen tap had run for several minutes that failed to capture the full potential for Pb exposure. We expected Pb exposure risks could be high in ETJ communities without water service because households relying on private wells typically do not have treatment systems capable of preventing Pb release from well components and household plumbing and fixtures (11). (Until 2014, water fixtures could contain up to 8% Pb and be declared "lead free" (12)). As a result, Stillo's project focused on Pb. Pb is a potent neurotoxin that can lead to irreversible cognitive damage in children (13, 14). In Flint, the prevalence of elevated blood Pb (defined at the time as ≥ 5 μg/dL) more than doubled during the water crisis, in some areas increasing to more than 15% (from a city-wide average of 2.4% before the crisis) (15).

Stillo recruited households from Wake County ETJ communities relying on private wells to participate in free water testing. He found high Pb concentrations in 28% of homes (see Figure 2. This fraction was comparable to the prevalence of elevated Pb in water in Flint, Michigan, during the water crisis. Among Flint's nine wards, Ward 5 had the highest risk of exposure to Pb, with elevated Pb (≥ 15 ppb) in 32% of homes (16). The second-most impacted neighborhoods were Wards 6 and 7, with 28% of homes exposed to elevated Pb, the same percentage as Stillo's BTC project uncovered in the ETJs of Wake County (16, 17). Unlike in Flint, however, no authority is responsible for monitoring Pb in drinking water in ETJs or for taking action when Pb concentrations are high. Residents of these areas will not be eligible for the types of legal compensation available to municipal residents who are harmed if the community water supply fails to discharge its duty to prevent exposure to Pb.

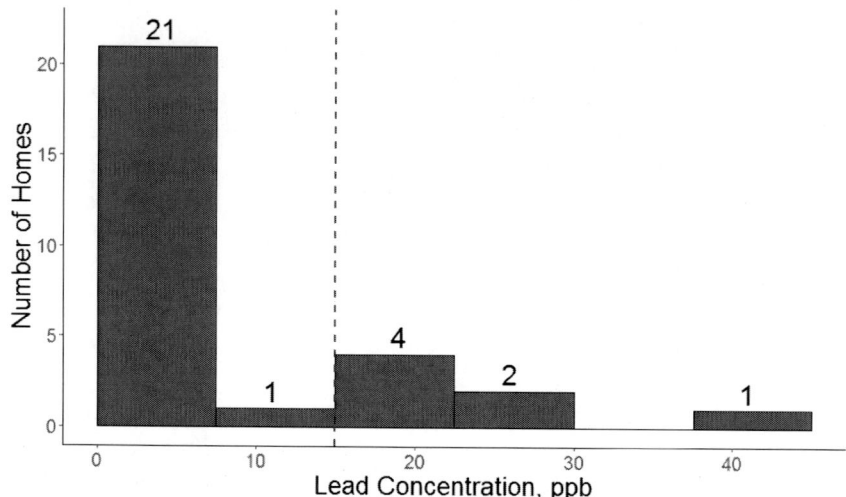

Figure 2. Frank Stillo's BTC project found that water in 7 of 29 (28%) of sampled homes in extraterritorial jurisdictions without community services exceeded the 15-ppb action level for Pb that community water systems must meet. This prevalence of elevated Pb in water was similar to that occurring in the most affected wards of Flint, Michigan, during the water crisis. Reproduced from (17).

BTC 2017–2018 and 2021–2022: Effects of water service inequities on blood lead

Participants in subsequent BTC cohorts built on Dr Stillo's research to demonstrate that increased risks of exposure to elevated Pb in private well water in Wake County ETJs, compared to in areas receiving community water service, is associated with adverse effects on children.

Allison Clonch, in the BTC 2017–2018 cohort, built a curated data set linking blood Pb data for 34,314 Wake County children to information on the children's water sources, characteristics of their household (age and value), and neighborhood demographics. She found that children served by community water systems had significantly lower blood Pb than children relying on private well water when controlling for demographic and socioeconomic factors (see Table 1) (18). A subsequent expansion of this work to include 59,483 children, completed after Ally's BTC project, confirmed these results (19).

Table 1. Factors influencing children's blood Pb levels in Wake County, NC (reproduced from (18))

Variables	B	p-value
Community Water System Access at Birth	-0.12	<0.0001
Year Tested	-0.092	<0.0001
Black Population Fraction	0.23	<0.0001
Home Value (Log10, US$)	-0.22	<0.0001
Gender	0.037	0.0059
Municipal Status	0.038	0.24
Hispanic Population Fraction	-0.085	0.44
Median Household Income	<0.0001	0.6
Age		
18 to 36 Months	0.13	<0.0001
36 to 54 Months	0.095	0.01
Over 54 Months	0.053	0.73
Year House Built		
1970 to 1950	-0.33	<0.0001
1970 to 1990	-0.41	<0.0001
1990 to 2000	-0.5	<0.0001
2000 to 2005	-0.55	<0.0001
After 2005	-0.44	<0.0001
N	34,314	

Alyson Alde, in the BTC 2021–2022 cohort, completed a field study to assess whether Ms. Clonch's finding that blood Pb is associated with Pb exposure from private wells could be confirmed through simultaneous collection of water and blood Pb samples. She (and other students) recruited 89 individuals in NC households relying on private wells water to participate. As reported in Ms. Alde's article in this issue, she found that Pb in private well water was indirectly associated with blood Pb through use of a water filter. Those that filtered their water had significantly lower (by 32%) blood Pb concentrations than those without water filters. She also found substantial racial disparities in access to a household water filter: 38% of African Americans had water filters, compared to 83% of those of other racial and ethnic groups.

Dr Michelle Del Rio, a post-doctoral scholar in the BTC 2021–2022 cohort, undertook a systematic literature review on demographic, social, economic, and environmental factors associated with Pb exposure to further advance understanding of the extent to which inequities in access to regulated community water supplies may affect overall Pb exposure. She used the results to develop a social-ecological model of Pb exposure risk that can guide future studies on the contribution of water source to longstanding racial disparities in children's blood Pb levels. The model (described in Dr Del Rio's article in this issue) and related follow-on research can help to design early intervention strategies and leverage more effectively the limited resources available to address childhood exposure to Pb.

Mentee outcomes

Participating in BTC helped shape the careers of all of these mentees. Frank Stillo's BTC project formed part of his PhD dissertation. The results (findings of elevated Pb in drinking water of many of the tested households) motivated him to study the effectiveness of risk communication and financial interventions to prevent Pb exposure in ETJ communities, the focus of the remaining chapters of his dissertation. He leveraged the knowledge he gained to secure a position as Project Scientist at Geosyntec Consultants, where his roles include risk assessment and communication and the development of community partnerships. Allison Clonch's epidemiologic analysis of associations between exclusion from community water service and children's blood Pb served as the basis for her MSPH thesis. The experience motivated her to shift from a focus on environmental science to pursue a PhD degree in epidemiology; she is currently a PhD student in the Department of Epidemiology at the University of Washington. Michelle Del Rio is using her BTC project to conceptualize a proposal to the National Institutes of Health for interventions to prevent cognitive damage from low-level exposure to Pb in children. Dr Del Rio recently accepted her first faculty position (Assistant Professor in the Department of Environmental and Occupational Health at Indiana University, Bloomington). This proposal will lay the foundation for her independent research program focused on breaking the entrenched cycle of disparities in exposure to Pb among U.S. children. Alyson Alde's BTC project became her master's thesis—the first in her family. She leveraged her field research experience to become a research scientist supporting projects on children's environmental health at the Indiana University, Bloomington, School of Public Health.

Spillover benefits to other students

The BTC mentees motivated other students (beyond the BTC program) to pursue related research:

- MS student Sidney Lockhart documented how exclusion from community water service affected activities of daily life in one ETJ community (20). She found that 65% of residents experienced failures of their private well at least once a year, leaving them with an insufficient quantity of water for bathing, handwashing, dishwashing, and doing laundry. More than three-quarters of residents wanted to be connected to the water supply for the neighboring town.
- MSPH student Julia Naman conducted qualitative research to identify structural factors perpetuating inequitable water and sanitation service access in ETJs (21). She interviewed 25 key informants including elected officials, health officials, water and sewer utility staff, and community members. She found that inadequate funding was the biggest barrier to extending services into ETJs. Decisionmakers also failed to consider the public health consequences of substandard water and sanitation services in evaluating costs of these services.
- PhD student Riley Mulhern investigated the effectiveness of off-the-shelf, low-cost, under-sink granular activated carbon filters as a short-term solution to prevent exposure to Pb and other contaminants in homes relying on private well water (22). He recruited 18 households with private wells (some in ETJs and others in rural areas) for an eight-month study in which participants received a free water filter, and water quality was monitored monthly. He demonstrated that the filters effectively removed 98% of Pb. Access to a filter decreased participants' perceived vulnerability to drinking water contamination. However, some participants' filters clogged, limiting water flow. The risk of clogging underscores that community water service is a preferable option in areas of sufficient population density (such as in ETJs), since community systems must control the turbidity and other characteristics of the water that make filters vulnerable to clogging of their water, which would prevent clogging in filters. In addition, the filters were unable to remove all of the potentially harmful bacteria and viruses from the water (23)—a concern that municipal water systems address by disinfecting the water before they distribute it.

Community benefits

The cumulative data from BTC and related projects helped one ETJ community successfully campaign for annexation into the adjacent town and connection to the town's water service. The Irongate Drive neighborhood, adjacent to Apex, NC, had long experienced water quantity and quality problems like those documented by my students' research. They had sought for years to connect to the Apex water supply, without success. BTC mentee Stillo recruited undergraduate students and other graduate students to assist the community by gathering data to present to the Apex town manager, mayor, and town council. These data helped persuade the town to extend water service into the Irongate neighborhood. Water service was established in spring and summer, 2020, enabling activities of daily home life like showering and doing laundry that most Americans take for granted. The community and my students also investigated whether the new water service would resolve the longstanding problems of elevated Pb in the drinking water. Led by master's student April Desclos, they found that Pb concentrations decreased by 70% on average after homes received community water service—a benefit resulting from the community system's corrosion control practices, which prevent the leaching of Pb from household plumbing and fixtures (24).

Conclusion

Participation in the BTC program has advanced my research on disparities in access to safe drinking water in the United States, helped launch the careers of several of my mentees, and delivered tangible benefits (a new water supply) for one historically African American community. Awareness of these disparities and a passion to eliminate them have spilled over to other students who did not participate directly in BTC. A primary goal for my academic career is to conduct research that leads to action to improve people's lives. The BTC program has been instrumental in realizing this goal.

Acknowledgments

I am grateful to Dr Jeffrey Engel for the motivation and support to pursue the work described here and for the many community members who participated.

Also, this work would have been impossible without the dedication of many students over more than a decade, including those mentioned in this paper and dozens of others. Also essential was funding to support the research. Funding was provided by a series of sponsors: the Robert Wood Johnson Foundation Mentored Research Scientist Development Program (award 70580); IBM Junior Faculty Development Award at the University of North Carolina at Chapel Hill; North Carolina Policy Collaboratory; National Science Foundation (award CMMI-2017207); and US Environmental Protection Agency Science to Achieve Results program (award RD-83927902).

References

[1] Owens DW. Extraterritorial jurisdiction for planning and development regulation. URL: https://www.sog.unc.edu/resources/legal-summaries/extraterritorial-jurisdiction-planning-and-development-regulation.

[2] Heaney C, Wing S, Wilson S. Public infrastructure disparities and the microbiological and chemical safety of drinking and surface water supplies in a community bordering a landfill. J Environ Health 2013;75(10):24–36.

[3] Musacchio A, Andrade L, O'Neill E, Re V, O'Dwyer J, Hynds PD. Planning for the health impacts of climate change: Flooding, private groundwater contamination and waterborne infection – A cross-sectional study of risk perception, experience and behaviours in the Republic of Ireland. Environ Res 2021;194:110707.

[4] Jasechko S, Perrone D. Global groundwater wells at risk of running dry. URL: https://www.science.org.

[5] MacDonald Gibson J, DeFelice N, Sebastian D, Leker H. Racial disparities in access to community water supply service in Wake County, North Carolina. Front Public Health Serv Syst Res 2014;3(3):6.

[6] Leker HG, MacDonald Gibson J. Relationship between race and community water and sewer service in North Carolina, USA. PLoS One 2018;13(3):1–19.

[7] Aiken C. Race as a factor in municipal underbounding. Anna Assoc Am Geographers 1987;77:564-79.

[8] Lichter DT, Parisi D, Grice SM, Taquino M. Municipal underbounding: Annexation and racial exclusion in small southern towns. Rural Sociol 2007;72(1):47–68.

[9] Durst NJ. Municipal annexation and the selective underbounding of colonias in Texas' Lower Rio Grande Valley. Environ Plan A 2014;46(7):1699–715.

[10] Heaney CD, Wing S, Wilson SM, Campbell RL, O'Shea S, Caldwell D, et al. Public infrastructure disparities and the microbiological and chemical safety of drinking and surface water supplies in a community bordering a landfill. J Environ Health 2013;75(10):24–36.

[11] Malecki KMC, Schultz AA, Severtson DJ, Anderson HA, VanDerslice JA. Private-well stewardship among a general population based sample of private well-owners. Sci Total Environ 2017;601–602:1533–43.

[12] US Congress. Reduction of Lead in Drinking Water Act. Washington, DC: US Congress, 2011.

[13] Lanphear BP, Hornung R, Khoury J, Baghurst P, Bellinger DC, Canfield RL, et al. Low-level environmental lead exposure and children's intellectual function: An international pooled analysis. Environ Health Perspect 2005;113(7):894–9.

[14] Mazumdar M, Bellinger DC, Gregas M, Abanilla K, Bacic J, Needleman HL. Low-level environmental lead exposure in childhood and adult intellectual function: a follow-up study. Environ Health 2011;10:24.

[15] Hanna-Attisha M, LaChance J, Sadler RC, Schnepp AC. Elevated blood lead levels in children associated with the Flint drinking water crisis: A spatial analysis of risk and public health response. Am J Public Health 2016;106(2):283–90.

[16] Hanna-Attisha M, Lachance J, Sadler RC, Schnepp AC. Elevated blood lead levels in children associated with the Flint drinking water crisis: a spatial analysis of risk and public health response. Am J Public Health 2016;106(2):283–90.

[17] Stillo FJ, MacDonald Gibson J. Racial disparities in access to municipal water supplies in the American South: Impacts on children's health. Int Public Health J 2018;10(3):309–23.

[18] Clonch A, Fisher Mi, MacDonald Gibson J. Water infrastructure and childhood blood lead levels: characterizing the effects of ex-clusion from municipal services in Wake County (NC, USA). Int J Child Health Hum Dev 2019;12(4):425-34.

[19] Gibson JM, Fisher M, Clonch A, MacDonald J, Cook P. Children drinking private well water have higher blood lead than those with city water. Proceed Natl Acad Sci 2020;117(29):16898–907.

[20] Lockhart S, Wood E, MacDonald Gibson J. Impacts of exclusion from municipal water service on water availability: a case study. New Solutions 2020;30(2):127–37.

[21] Naman JM, Gibson JM. Disparities in water and sewer services in North Carolina: An analysis of the decision-making process. Am J Public Health 2015;105(10):e20-6.

[22] Mulhern R, Gibson JM. Under-sink activated carbon water filters effectively remove lead from private well water for over six months. Water (Switzerland) 2020;12(12):3584.

[23] Mulhern R, Stallard M, Zanib H, Stewart J, Sozzi E, MacDonald Gibson J. Are carbon water filters safe for private wells? Evaluating the occurrence of microbial indicator organisms in private well water treated by point-of-use activated carbon block filters. Int J Hyg Environ Health 2021;238:113852.

[24] Desclos, A. Evaluation of drinking water contamination in a peri-urban neighborhood after connection to municipal water service. Master's thesis. Chapel Hill, NC: University of North Carolina, 2021.

Chapter 3

Break the Cycle: Challenges and impacts in Latin American communities

Patricia M Valenzuela[1,*], MD, MSc
M Rosario Moore[1], MD, MSc
María Soledad Matus[2], MD
María I Eugenin[1], MD
Alejandra Nuñez-Palma[1], MD
and Javiera Martínez-Gutiérrez[3,4], MD, MPH

[1]Department of Pediatrics, Facultad de Medicina, Pontificia Universidad Católica de Chile, Santiago, Chile
[2]Pediatric Emergency Department, Department of Pediatrics, Clínica Alemana, Santiago, Chile
[3]Department of Family Medicine, Facultad de Medicina, Pontificia Universidad Católica de Chile, Santiago, Chile
[4]Department of General Practice, Faculty of Dentistry, Medicine, and Health Services, School of Medicine, University of Melbourne, Melbourne, Australia

Abstract

The Break the Cycle (BTC) program was developed to promote quality research focusing on underserved communities, for example covering prevalent issues that affect underserved communities in Latin America. Chilean studies: Three studies were developed with BTC support. The students were pediatric residents whose research topics were discussed

---

[*] ***Correspondence:*** Patricia M Valenzuela, MD, Associate Professor, Department of Pediatrics, Facultad de Medicina, Pontificia Universidad Católica de Chile, Santiago, Chile, 362 Diagonal Paraguay, 8th floor, Santiago 8330077, Chile. Email: pvalenzc@uc.cl.

In: Environmental Health Disparities
Editors: I. Leslie Rubin and Joav Merrick
ISBN: 979-8-89113-487-4
© 2024 Nova Science Publishers, Inc.

with their Chilean mentors and the BTC team. The main results of these studies were the following: 1) Identification of increased awareness of indoor environmental risk factors for pediatric respiratory diseases in an underserved community: 50 families, 32% of children had past illnesses (87.5% asthma); 24% reported smoking happening in the home; 62% had animals living indoors. 2) Screening for autism; Community perspectives: We screened 200 children (16 to 30 months of age) with the M-CHAT and M-CHAT follow-up interview (MC-FUI) in middle-low and very low socioeconomic and vulnerable communities. 22% screened positive; 11.4% of them continued to be at risk after the MC-FUI. Two children were confirmed for ASD. 3) Measuring parenting dimensions and social and prosocial abilities in adolescents living in vulnerable families. 120 adolescents reported that most caregivers had an authoritative parenting style. There was a correlation between high parenting demandingness and monitoring, with high prosocial skills among adolescents. Conclusions: The BTC program created great opportunities for students and mentors to improve and expand their research by including the social determinants of health. Being more aware of social disparities helped them to focus on finding ways to break the cycle.

Introduction

Latin America and the Caribbean have made substantial progress in economic and social development during the last 20 years, yet it is still one of the regions in the world with the most inequalities. Children and adolescents are very vulnerable and are uniquely impacted by these disparities; our perspectives as pediatricians and pediatric residents give us particular interest in addressing these public health issues in clinical practice, as researchers, and as academicians.

As an example, in Latin America, there are currently 82 million people without access to basic sanitation services, (representing approximately 12% of the Latin American population) and 20 million with no proper access to drinking water (1). Although lower than the staggering worldwide average of almost 50% of the population without sanitation services worldwide, it also follows the pattern of disparities affecting mostly rural and underserved areas (2). Regarding domestic violence, 63% of children under 15 years of age experience either physical and/or psychologically violent discipline at home, and 1 out of 10 children are alone or under the care of another child, every day. The adolescent homicide rate is five times higher in Latin America and the Caribbean, compared to the global average (3).

Inappropriate food supply and the consumption of processed foods and drinks have made Latin American children victims of obesity. In 2020, UNICEF and the World Bank estimated that 4 million children were overweight. This number represents 7.5% of Latin American children, compared to 5.7% of children worldwide (4).

In Chile, infant mortality rates have shown an important decrease during the last fifty years (5, 6) as a result of the development of national health programs, such as infant nutrition, immunization, acute respiratory management, and improvement of the sanitary conditions all down and across the country. However, these important advances have not benefited all regions and social groups in the country in the same way. There are still big differences in mortality rate and quality of life between urban, more educated groups compared with underprivileged and remote communities. Infant mortality in Chile is 7.2/1,000 on average, and yet, it is as high as 8.6/1,000 in the region of La Araucania, where most of the indigenous populations live, and 9.7/1,000 in Aysen, one of the most remote regions in the country (7).

During the last thirty years the poverty rate in Chile has declined significantly, but the difference of income between the poorest and the richest has not declined at the same rate. Low income in a country like Chile not only means less purchasing power; it also means less access to quality education, fewer options for medical care, inadequate dwellings, and higher exposure to violence, among others. So, while the focus nowadays is on poverty rate, little is said about multidimensional poverty, a concept that involves education, health, social welfare, work, living space, social cohesion of communities, etc. Obviously, in Chile there are still important inequalities in underserved communities (8).

When child health professionals have been confronted with these inequalities, in real life patients, it has been impossible to remain oblivious, especially knowing there was so much that could be done to support these underprivileged communities. As pediatricians in Chile, seeing what it means to our patients, especially to a child or adolescent, to belong to a vulnerable community, was probably the main motivation for us to focus our attention on how to break the cycle of disparities. A big question was, 'How to start?' What could we do to have some kind of impact in these communities? The Break the Cycle program became the perfect starting point, as it gave us the opportunity to transform ideas into projects, and projects into actual change for the better.

Break the Cycle: A program to focus on targeting health disparities in our child and adolescent populations

The Break the Cycle (BTC) program was developed almost two decades ago to promote quality research focusing on social, economic, and environmental factors and their impact on children's health. The aim was to encourage young researchers to get involved in this area, and to promote leadership among students in participating and sharing their ideas on building a community of health professionals that would be empowered to think about solutions, focus their research, and create awareness of these societal problems.

Today, students and their mentors are selected through a competitive process from all over the world to participate in a rigorous program that entails monthly meetings with the rest of the group of mentors and students to launch new ideas and troubleshoot research problems encountered along the way. Students are required to present their methods and findings under the close supervision of a world-renowned group of faculty advisors.

The mentees are also required to present to a panel of experts and their fellow mentees from around the world at a meeting in the United States. The program ends with the publication of their work in peer reviewed international journals.

Throughout the years, Break the Cycle studies have covered a broad range of health problems, addressing some of the most prevalent issues that affect our underserved communities in Latin America. Some of the topics addressed have been: Maternal health in remote indigenous villages (Guatemala); Indoor risk factors/pollution and respiratory symptoms (Chile); Obesity prevention (Mexico); MCHAT for Autism Spectrum Disorders screening (Chile); Violence against children and youth prevention (Mexico); Predictors of completed childhood vaccination (Bolivia); Protecting children from harmful environmental exposures (Puerto Rico); A new health surveillance system for pregnant women (Brazil); Nurturing care and childhood development in low-income communities (Paraguay); and Cultivating social and prosocial abilities along adolescent and parenting dimensions (Chile).

All of these studies have targeted different social determinants of health. Because childhood is a dynamic process of growth and development, children are uniquely vulnerable to harmful determinants than other populations. The impact on children's health in disadvantaged communities is even greater since the risks are often cumulative, resulting in wider health disparities. The studies mentioned above have undoubtedly been great contributions to the communities where they were carried out. The risk factors identified, and the validated screening tests and surveillance tools have been crucial to carrying out interventions that directly benefit them, helping to break the cycle of children's health disparities in Latin America.

Likewise, in our experience this program has been a great opportunity for students and mentors to focus their research on emphasizing the social determinants of health. Traditionally, medicine has focused its research mainly on the biological aspects of a problem. With BTC, the research topics have changed, now expanding from just looking at the biology of a health problem, to including the social and economic inequalities which can cause them, and interfere with their resolution. The students have grown in knowledge, and have opened their minds to a more comprehensive way of understanding health problems; they are more aware of social disparities and are able to focus their research on looking for answers that could help to break the cycle of inequality and disease.

Chilean case studies: Changing the way we teach, the medical curriculum, and the impact on our population

Pediatric residents at Pontificia Universidad Católica de Chile are required to complete a research project and publish it before graduating. It is a large part of their overall evaluation, and they have three years to complete it during their residency. For example, the following three students participated concomitantly in the BTC program, further empowering them, and providing them with excellent tools and opportunities for their final projects.

Case 1. Indoor environmental risk factors for pediatric respiratory diseases in an underserved community in Santiago, Chile (9)

In 2012-2013, Maria Soledad Matus carried out her research project within the BTC program. This allowed her to not only help an underserved community, but to provide valuable information regarding indoor environmental risk factors to the families and the health care teams caring for them. Participating in the BTC program was a unique and very enriching experience for everyone who was part of this project and, above all, for the families with whom we worked.

As a pediatrics resident, with her involvement in BTC, she was able to broaden her vision about what it meant to be a pediatrician, further strengthening her belief that prevention and health promotion are fundamental when working directly with the community.

Environmental pediatrics was not an area that had been thoroughly explored in the pediatric curriculum. Conducting this research allowed both Maria Soledad and her supervisors to increase the focus on the importance of teaching that subject, and conducting good quality research in that direction.

The guidance BTC provides on research methods prompted a rigorous search of existing literature on the topic, and encouraged the researcher to embed herself in the evidence and theories behind environmental pediatrics. For the first time, she felt she had to use and put into practice all her newly acquired research skills. Furthermore, the need to record her methods and results in a systematic process, and to write it up in an academic paper, in English, which was not her native language, was a very strenuous, useful, and rewarding challenge.

To select our research topic, we knew we wanted to have a real impact on the health of underserved communities. We learned that there were many environmental risk factors described in the international literature, and that many of them were not being identified as harmful factors for health in our communities. This became a strong motivator for overcoming these challenges, and an opportunity to inform families and the healthcare teams about environmental risk factors and to implement ways to prevent disease.

Respiratory diseases are the first cause of pediatric hospitalizations and multiple consultations in health centers in Chile (10-12). Household pollution is one of the main risk factors for acute respiratory infection, particularly in poor areas and crowded homes.

Based on the above, we conducted a descriptive study to identify indoor risk factors for respiratory symptoms in an underserved community in Santiago, Chile. The study included both quantitative and qualitative methodologies to characterize the presence of environmental risk factors, as well as to ascertain the knowledge and attitudes of the children's caregivers towards pollution and its effects on health.

The population studied included 50 families. Thirty two percent of the children had histories of past illnesses, and, of these, 87.5% had asthma. Twenty-four percent of the families reported that at least one person in the home smoked, and 62% had animals living inside the house. Liquefied gas was identified as the most common primary source of heating energy.

Participants reported the presence of air pollution subjectively throughout their homes.

We concluded that this community was exposed to numerous indoor environmental risk factors related to respiratory diseases. There was a lack of knowledge among the children's caregivers on the ill effects of pollution on children's health. Addressing this issue with the community was crucial as prevention of exposure can be one of the most effective ways to protect children's health, and since healthy indoor environments, especially home environments, are often controllable by adult behaviors (smoking, cooking, ventilation, etc.).

Thanks to this work, families were enabled to identify indoor risk factors, discussed solutions to avoid them, and were able to involve the community in participating in disease prevention, and empower the families with their self-care.

Carrying out this environmental pediatric study in direct collaboration with families complemented Maria Soledad's training as a specialist developing her ability to extend beyond solely medical practice with the patients, to including information regarding their entire families and environment. Including the families in the research effort provides ongoing benefits for all.

Case 2. Screening for autism in Santiago Chile: Community perspectives (13)

During 2013-2014, we explored preliminary screening for autism spectrum disorders (ASD) using M-CHAT in two underserved Chilean communities at a time when no such screening existed in our country. ASD prevalence has increased in the last 30 years and requires prompt detection to improve children's developmental outcomes. They were not easily diagnosed in primary care settings as they usually required child development assessments which were not easily accessible. Maria Ignacia Eugenin, at that time a first-year pediatric resident, took on this project as her thesis. She used the M-CHAT and M-CHAT follow-up interview with 200 children (16 to 30 months of age) in two medical centers (in low and very low socioeconomic and vulnerable communities). 22% of the children screened positive initially, and 11.4% (five patients in total) continued to screen at-risk after a follow-up interview. Of those five patients, three attended a formal evaluation afterwards, and ASD was confirmed in two. For these two patients, early diagnosis of ASD probably improved their future outcomes since they were promptly referred for appropriate evaluations and therapies (14).

Part of this study was also qualitative, with focus groups carried out with parents in both communities. The results were very interesting, and valuable insights into the understanding of this screening tool were shared in the Chilean population. In summary, three main topics were encountered from the parents´ perspectives: 1) the perception of ignorance about ASD: the overall knowledge about ASD in those communities was very low; 2) that families were as important as healthcare professionals for making the diagnosis since they probably know their child best; 3) and many mothers identified play as a way of stimulating psychomotor development. Additionally, particularly in the very vulnerable population, mothers described that as they read the questionnaire, they also learned and paid more attention to the developmental aspects of their children that they did not know about before (for example, one mother mentioned she had never paid attention to whether or not her child used direct eye contact).

Part of the group of investigators moved forward and carried out a cultural adaptation in 2017 (15), and then published a formal validation in 2019 of the M-CHAT-R/F in the Chilean population (16). As a result, the M-CHAT-R/F was incorporated as a formal recommendation in the Chilean Health Ministry Guidelines for Well-Child-Care Visits (17). These guidelines are used in primary care throughout the public healthcare system in the entire country (which is 2,653 miles long and geographically complex), directly benefiting the most vulnerable Chilean populations. The technical guidelines provide not only guidance in good-quality care, but also promote a context of equity, ensuring that the care of both boys and girls, regardless of their socio demographic conditions, receive the same universal minimum health benefits throughout the country.

This is a clear example of how a body of research that was done rigorously with the help of the program, targeted a particularly vulnerable population, tested and validated the right intervention, and yielded a public policy in a short period of time. This outcome showcases the power and relevance of BTC in our region.

Case 3. Measuring parenting dimensions and social and prosocial abilities in adolescents from vulnerable families in Chile (18)

During 2019-2020 Alejandra Nuñez-Palma carried out her research project within the BTC program. It took place in one of the most underserved communities in Chile, and was designed to evaluate the impact on the development of important skills for children of the interactions between the parents and these children. Surveys of adolescents from this community were used which asked the participants to describe the parenting styles of their caregivers from the adolescent's point of view; to describe their own social and prosocial skills, and to evaluate whether or not there was a correlation between them. We applied three validated questionnaires: one for parenting dimensions, one for social skills, and one for prosocial skills ("prosocial behavior is defined as the voluntary behavior that seeks the benefit of other people").

One hundred twenty adolescents took part in this research, of whom 52% were female. We found that almost all the caregivers were described as highly demanding but also as highly responsive, so their parenting style was regarded as authoritative. Regarding social skills, 72% of the participants were classified as moderately skilled socially, and only 10% as socially skilled. As to prosocial skills, 38.7% were considered to be prosocially impaired, and 37.8% prosocially skilled. We also found a correlation between high parenting demandingness and monitoring with high prosocial skills among the adolescents.

Alejandra was highly motivated to conduct this research as she had been required to do a rotation in her last year of practice as a medical student in a primary health center in one of the poorest communities in Chile. One of the things that drew her attention was the way in which parents and children interacted. It seemed that parents were more authoritarian than those she had seen in other communities. She wondered if this had some kind of impact on the development of the children. It was not until she heard about the Break the Cycle Program that she felt it was possible to answer that question. By partnering with the schools and healthcare centers, we were able to bring the community together, promote awareness, and provide problem oriented education for caregivers and educators.

BTC in teaching (Patricia M Valenzuela)

I have been the primary mentor for these three projects for the last 10 years. As a Latin American pediatrician, educator, and researcher, it's been very rewarding to offer BTC as an incredible opportunity for my students to focus on the local problems in our communities with a global health perspective.

From the student's perspective, BTC has been a unique opportunity for personal development and accomplishment, particularly in Latin American countries where access to top tier academics is not an opportunity for everyone. Mentees were able to participate with real time feedback by experts in scheduled and continuing meetings from the inception to the completion of their projects. They were able to share their projects and learn from other students and professors. The opportunities for advancing their research, overcoming language-barriers, having networking experiences, traveling, experiencing camaraderie with other students, and achieving overall personal growth were endless. Back at home, the students were recognized for the excellency of their work at their university. Their projects and publications were part of their post-graduate theses, and I am proud to say that they won "Best fellow" and various other research awards.

Moreover, my experience of participating in BTC during these years has had an important influence on my way of teaching. In the context of a new curriculum developed at the Faculty of Medicine, I had the opportunity to work with a multidisciplinary team to design and implement a new course for first-year students of Medicine. This course promotes the early contact of students with patients and their environment. Many studies have shown that early contact with patients by medical students has shown benefits for learning and developing skills and transversal competencies that will be useful in their future professional practices. Important topics addressed in our course are: professionalism, social responsibility, teamwork, and health promotion and prevention among others. The students learn about social determinants and their relationship to the health of individuals, families, and communities; aspects of justice and equity in health care, identification of the scope of action at the primary level of care in the Chilean health system; recognition of the role of the various health agents within the team, and their contributions to health care. The course incorporated student-centered learning strategies using innovative pedagogical resources. Students have the opportunity to perform a service activity with promotion and promoting prevention in an underserved community, using Service-Learning methodology, in which knowledge and skills acquired in the course are applied. Our hope is that all these experiences and skills facilitated by the course, will help them develop a sense of social responsibility that will make for integral and wholesome health care professionals.

Students' reflections and career pathways

Maria Soledad Matus, MD, Deputy Chief of the Pediatric Emergency Department, Clinica Alemana, Santiago, Chile: Participating in Break the Cycle has been one of the most enriching experiences in my training as a pediatrician. Working with mentors and teachers on a monthly basis throughout the project, and learning new methodologies, made me want to be an educator as well as a practitioner, and after my pediatrics residency, I completed a teaching certificate. I have been teaching undergraduate medicine, pediatrics, and supervising emergency residents for the past eight years. This has been a major area of academic development, and it has provided multiple satisfactions in my career.

Working on my research project with Break the Cycle gave me the opportunity to present my project to an international forum for the first time, which clearly marked a milestone in my development as a student and as a medical doctor. Being able to meet people from different backgrounds allowed me to realize that there are many of us who want to make changes and contribute to breaking the cycle of health disparities.

I currently work as the deputy chief of the pediatric emergency department of one of the largest pediatric emergency rooms in the country and, it is here that I have chosen to continue to engage with the community, especially in terms of disease prevention and health promotion, which was one of the most important lessons I learned with BTC. Finally, I am very thankful for the opportunity to have participated in BTC, and I want to encourage future young researchers to continue on this path of promoting health equity for all children in Latin America.

Maria Ignacia Eugenin, MD, Children with Special Healthcare Needs Specialist: BTC was an amazing opportunity for me as a pediatric resident. I was given the opportunity to work with my mentors, and received invaluable guidance on the development of my research project. This was also a great life experience, as it was my first professional travel opportunity. I participated in person at the BTC conference, met outstanding people, and built connections, and I also had the chance to visit top of the line ASD centers, and the CDC building.

The theme of my project sparked my interest in working with children with various developmental needs. Upon graduating, I joined the Complex Child Care Unit at my hospital, and the Down Syndrome Center in our University, and have been working there ever since. This program has grown rapidly, as the incidence of children with special healthcare needs is on the rise worldwide, and I am proud to say that our group probably has the most experience nationwide. A great percentage of my patients has ASD or a dual diagnosis with Down syndrome, and I particularly value and enjoy working with these families. Looking back, it is moving to see how a particular project heavily influenced my career choice, and I am infinitely grateful for it.

Alejandra Nuñez-Palma, MD, Pediatric Cardiology Resident: Taking part in BTC was a very fulfilling experience for me. It not only provided me with very useful and important research tools, but also gave me the opportunity of being guided and supported by very qualified and caring staff through the process of planning and carrying out my project. I got to know students from other parts of the world, and learned about their own very interesting projects. It made me see other aspects of the same problem, perspectives that are far from my area of expertise. I learned about gentrification, about environmental justice, lead dust, and much more. It helped me realize that the problems that all these communities have to face are essentially very similar.

Currently, I am a Resident in Pediatric Cardiology, starting my last year. When I finish, I will be working in a public hospital for chronically ventilated children. These are very vulnerable children who face not only grave health problems, but also serious social conditions, and abandonment.

I have been appointed to start a new Department of Cardiology at the hospital in order to widen our scope to include children with congenital heart diseases. It is also our dream to start a Cardiopulmonary Rehabilitation Program to improve these children's quality of life.

From having a single question in my brain to organizing and conducting proper research, taking part in BTC gave me the opportunity to get involved in a vulnerable community, talk to the children, adolescents, and teachers, and realize that I wanted to do something meaningful for vulnerable children. Since then, I have steered my career in that direction. I am grateful for the opportunity that BTC gave me to see that there are people who care about vulnerable children and work for a better future for them.

Acknowledgments

Finally, we would like to extend our gratitude to Dr Leslie Rubin and his team of faculty members at Emory University. We have had the privilege of participating in these three different BTC programs across the years, which has created a tremendous opportunity for our students, us, as mentors, our university, and finally our community. We are sure BTC will continue to enable high quality, impactful research in Latin America, and we are excited about continuing to support future generations of Latin American researchers through this program. We hope many other researchers in our region join this important initiative to Break the Cycle of Children's Environmental Health Disparities to promote health equity for all children.

References

[1] UNICEF. Children live in a safe and clean environment. .URL: https://www.unicef.org/lac/en/children-live-safe-and-clean-environment.
[2] World Bank. Sanitation overview: Development news, research, data. URL: https://www.worldbank.org/en/topic/sanitation.
[3] UNICEF. Children in Latin America and the Caribbean. URL: https://www.unicef.org/lac/en/children-latin-america-and-caribbean.
[4] UNICEF. 3 in 10 children and adolescents in Latin America and the Caribbean have overweight. URL: https://www.unicef.org/lac/en/press-releases/3-in-10-children-and-adolescents-in-latin-america-and-the-caribbean-have-overweight.
[5] Kaempffer A, Medina E. Mortalidad infantil reciente en Chile: Exitos y desafíos. Rev Chil Pediatr 2006;77(5):492-500.
[6] World Bank Statistics 2020. Infant Mortality in Chile. URL: https://datos.bancomundial.org/share/widget?indicators=SP.DYN.IMRT.IN&locations=CL.
[7] Ministerio de Salud, Chile. Departamento de Estadísticas e Información en Salud | Mortalidad infantil y sus componentes, por Región y Comuna de residencia de la madre. Chile. URL: https://informesdeis.minsal.cl/SASVisualAnalytics/?reportUri=%2Freports%2Freports%2F4013de47-a3c2-47b8-8547-075525e4f819&sectionIndex=0&sso_guest=true&reportViewOnly=true&reportContextBar=false&sas-welcome=false.
[8] Fuentealba GL. Mortalidad infantil y pobreza en Chile: estudio ecológico a nivel comunal. Master of Public Health Thesis. Santiago, Chile: Pontificia Universidad Católica de Chile, 2021. URL: https://repositorio.uc.cl/handle/11534/57916.
[9] Matus MS, Sanchez T, Martinez-Gutierrez J, Cerda J, Molina H, Valenzuela PM. Indoor environmental risk factors for pediatric respiratory diseases in an underserved community in Santiago, Chile. Int J Child Health Hum Dev 2014;7(3):249-58.

[10] Ministerio de Salud, Gobierno de Chile | Guía clínica infección respiratoria aguda baja de manejo ambulatorio de 5 años. Santiago:Health Ministry, 2013. URL: https://www.minsal.cl/portal/url/item/7220fdc4341244a9e04001011f0113b9.pdf.

[11] Astudillo P, Mancilla P, Olmos C, Reyes A. Epidemiología de las consultas pediátricas respiratorias en Santiago de Chile desde 1993 a 2009. Rev Panam Salud Publica 2012;32(1):56-61.

[12] Barría M, Calvo M. Factores asociados a infecciones respiratorias dentro de los primeros tres meses de vida. Rev Chil Pediatr 2008;79(3):281-89.

[13] Eugenin MI, Moore R, Martinez-Gutierrez J, Perez CA, Valenzuela PM. Screening for autism in Santiago Chile: Community perspectives. Int J Child Adolesc Health 2015;8(4):439-48.

[14] Whitehouse AJO, Varcin KJ, Pillar S, Billingham W, Alvares GA, Barbaro J, et al. Effect of preemptive intervention on developmental outcomes among infants showing early signs of autism: A randomized clinical trial of outcomes to diagnosis. *JAMA Pediatr* 2021;175(11):e213298. doi:10.1001/jamapediatrics.2021.3298.

[15] Coelho-Medeiros M, Bronstein J, Aedo K, Pereira J, Arraño V, Perez CA, et al. Relevancia de la adaptación cultural en la validación del M-CHAT-R/F como instrumento de tamizaje precoz para autismo. Rev Chil Pediatr 2017;88(6):822-23.

[16] Coelho-Medeiros M, Bronstein J, Aedo K, Pereira J, Arraño V, Perez CA, et al. M-CHAT-R/F Validation as a screening tool for early detection in children with autism spectrum disorder. Rev Chil Pediatr 2019;90(5):492-99.

[17] Ministerio de Salud, Chile | Norma Técnica para la Supervisión de Salud Integral de niños y niñas de 0 a 9 años en APS. Santiago: Ministry of Health, 2021. URL: https://www.minsal.cl/ministerio-de-salud-presenta-actualizacion-de-norma-tecnica-para-la-supervision-de-salud-integral-de-ninos-y-ninas-de-0-a-9-anos-en-aps/.

[18] Núñez-Palma A, Vergara-López M, Seguel R, Pérez-Valenzuela J, Lozano J, Martínez-Gutiérrez J, Valenzuela PM. Measuring parenting dimensions and social and prosocial abilities in adolescents from vulnerable families in Chile. Int Public Health J 2021;13(4):415-29.

Chapter 4

Factors influencing inequities in lead exposure in United States children: A systematic review

Michelle Del Rio*, MPH, PhD, and Jacqueline MacDonald Gibson, PhD

Department of Environmental and Occupational Health, Indiana University Bloomington, Bloomington, Indiana, United States of America
Department of Civil, Construction, and Environmental Engineering, North Carolina State University, Raleigh, North Carolina, United States of America

Abstract

Although US policies to limit lead (Pb) release into the environment have substantially decreased children's blood Pb concentrations over the past four decades, more than a million children are still exposed to harmful Pb levels. A social-ecological model (SEM) of childhood Pb exposure may help public health professionals and government officials prevent these exposures by identifying the combinations of individual and social environmental factors that have resisted previous Pb exposure control policies and programs. To develop such an SEM, we conducted a systematic review of studies of children's blood Pb in the United States published since 2005. Information on risk factors for Pb exposure was extracted from each article. Identified risk factors were then grouped into the five levels of an SEM: intrapersonal, interpersonal, institutional, community, and public policy. In total, the review identified 75 peer-reviewed studies of children's Pb exposure in the United States since 2005. The review revealed that while child blood Pb levels have declined

---

* *Correspondence:* Michelle Del Rio, MPH, PhD, Assistant professor, Department of Environmental and Occu-pational Health, Indiana University Bloomington, 1025 E 7th St, Bloomington, IN 47405, United States. E-mail: midelrio@iu.edu.

In: Environmental Health Disparities
Editors: I. Leslie Rubin and Joav Merrick
ISBN: 979-8-89113-487-4
© 2024 Nova Science Publishers, Inc.

over time, inequities of Pb exposure persist among Non-Hispanic Black, migrant, and low-income children. Mixed effects were reported for Hispanic/Latinx/Mexican-American populations, with some studies finding these groups were at higher risk and others showing lower risks. Surprisingly, some studies found higher blood Pb in children over age 5 than in younger children, though the reverse was generally true. Findings reveal new opportunities to target exposure prevention programs at the intrapersonal, institutional, community, and policy levels. Well-controlled studies of the effectiveness of interventions at each level are needed to guide future policymaking.

Keywords: childhood, children, lead exposure, lead poisoning, risk factors, United States

Introduction

United States (US) policies since the 1970s have substantially decreased children's exposure to lead (Pb). These include bans or limitations on Pb in house paint, gasoline, food cans, plumbing materials, and drinking water (1). Nonetheless, children's exposure to Pb remains an important public health problem. A recent study estimated that 287,292 US children ages 0–4 years and another 588,995 ages 5–9 years had blood Pb levels (BLLs) greater than or equal to 5 µg/dL (which was, until recently, the recommended threshold for identifying children at higher risk from Pb) (2). For multiple reasons, the true number of children at risk is likely much higher. First, recent research has demonstrated that no level of Pb exposure is safe (3). For example, multiple studies have linked BLLs below 2.5 µg/dL with lower scholarly performance and behavioral problems in children (4–7). Second, the estimate excludes children older than age 9 years. Third, the cross-sectional design of the data on which the estimate is based (the National Health and Nutrition Examination Survey) disregards the potential temporal variation in Pb exposure (8) and absorption that can arise from changes in social, economic, and environmental factors throughout childhood. As a result, it is likely that far more than one million US children experience adverse effects from Pb exposure. The consequences of these preventable exposures extend well beyond the affected children and their families. For example, one study estimated that due to the cognitive damage in exposed children, every 1% increase in the tonnage of Pb emitted to air in US cities 22 years prior, increased the rate of aggravated assault during the time period 1972–2007 by 0.46% (9).

The potential size of the at-risk population and wide-reaching social consequences underscore the need for updated policies and other interventions to prevent children's Pb exposure. Existing policies and prevention programs may need to be strengthened, and new approaches may be needed to address entrenched problems of Pb exposure that have escaped previous control efforts and that are below levels previously not considered hazardous.

This paper advances the development of a social ecological model (SEM) of Pb exposure risk to inform Pb policy and program design. The SEM, first conceived by McLeroy et al. in 1988, recognizes that poor health cannot be improved by individual behaviors and actions alone. As conceptualized by McLeroy et al., the SEM consists of five nested levels:

- Intrapersonal factors, which are characteristics and behaviors specific to the individual (including health and developmental history, knowledge, and behaviors).
- Interpersonal factors, describing an individual's family and other primary social groups.
- Institutional factors, referring to "social institutions with organizational characteristics . . . and rules and regulations for operation" (10).
- Community factors, encompassing "relationships among organizations, institutions, and informal networks with defined boundaries" (10).
- Policies, including local, state, and national laws and regulations.

Since first proposed by McLeroy, SEMs have been used to conceptualize disease prevention and health promotion programs targeting a range of health risk factors, ranging from folic acid deficiencies to alcohol consumption. To our knowledge, however, an SEM model of childhood Pb exposure prevention has not been developed.

To construct the SEM model, we conducted a systematic literature review to capture current knowledge of factors associated with children's Pb exposure in the United States. Because policies established over the past several decades have dramatically altered Pb exposure patterns, we focus on research published since 2005. We used the literature review results to identify processes operating at each of the SEM model's five levels that may be contributing to Pb exposures not sufficiently prevented by previous policies and interventions.

Methods

The systematic review followed protocols set by the Preferred Reporting Items for Systematic Reviews and Analyses (PRISMA) (11). We submitted the systematic review to the PROSPERO international database for systematic reviews in the health and social care (12) (submitted in January 2022).

Search criteria

Prior to searching for studies, the Medical Subject Headings (MeSH) was reviewed to identify potential search terms. Only one MeSH term, "lead poisoning," was relevant. We used this term along with the keywords "lead exposure," "child," "US" and "factor" to search for articles of interest in PubMed. The search was conducted between January and March 2022. Articles were uploaded to COVIDENCE, a web-based software for screening articles for systematic reviews (13).

Inclusion criteria

Studies were selected for full-text review if they were published between 2005 and March 30, 2022; included children and/or adolescent populations (up to 18 years of age); were conducted in the United States; and measured child BLLs. Studies not reporting measured BLLs were excluded because BLLs are indicative of the most recent exposure and are used to guide clinical interventions. The review included all BLLs (no concentration cut points), whether from arm (venous) or finger stick (capillary) blood collection methods, analyzed using LeadCare devices or laboratory tests (such as from gas furnace atomic absorption spectrometry (GFAAS) or inductively coupled plasma mass spectrometry (ICPMS)). We excluded review articles, editorials, and non-peer-reviewed reports.

Table 1. Inclusion and exclusion criteria used to screen studies

Inclusion criteria	Exclusion criteria
• Children (18 years and under) • Population living in the U.S. 50 states • Blood Pb measurement of exposure • Published between January 1, 2005, and March 30, 2022	• Included adults or pregnant persons only • Measurement of exposure was not blood Pb • Published before 2005 • Editorials, reports, and review papers • Population living outside of U.S. 50 states and in U.S. territories

Screening and data extraction

Two independent reviewers first screened titles and abstracts for all of the identified studies. Each reviewer voted on whether the study met the inclusion criteria in Table 1 and should be advanced to full-text review. Disagreements were resolved through re-review and discussion.

For each retained study, the reviewers extracted the study year, location, purpose, and sample size; age range of participating children; summary statistics for measured BLLs; and factors associated with measured BLLs. Population-weighted means and medians were calculated by study year (with the mid-point of the study time period used in studies reporting data across multiple years). For each potential factor influencing Pb exposure assessed in the study, the direction of effect on BLL (positive or negative) and measure of significance (significant or insignificant) were noted. A positive direction meant that the factor was associated with higher BLLs. A negative direction meant that the factor was associated with lower BLLs. The measure of significance was based on univariate or multivariate statistical analysis results, where p-values ≤ 0.05 were considered significant. For some articles (4/75), significance was based on the author's statement of significance in the text.

Risk factor analysis

To provide qualitative information about the extent to which various risk factors have been studied and the consistency (or inconsistency) of findings across studies, we used a vote-counting technique adopted from previous systematic reviews (14, 15). Each study reporting on a given factor was assigned one vote based on the direction of the effect and measure of significance. When the direction of a factor was not clear, the vote was divided between negative and positive in the corresponding direction.

SEM development

Factors were organized into the five levels of the SEM: intrapersonal, interpersonal, organizational, community, and policy. Some factors may fit in two or more SEM levels, but for this review, we assigned each factor to only the SEM level we deemed most relevant. Results were used to diagram a proposed SEM of children's Pb exposure.

Results

The PubMed search located 1,134 studies; an additional two studies were identified through consultations with subject-matter experts. Of these, 75 met the inclusion criteria (see Figure 1). The number of studies published per year ranged between 1 and 9, with the years 2017 and 2022 having the most studies (see Figure 2). It appears there was a time trend that focused on Pb exposure increased after the Flint water crisis (2014–2016).

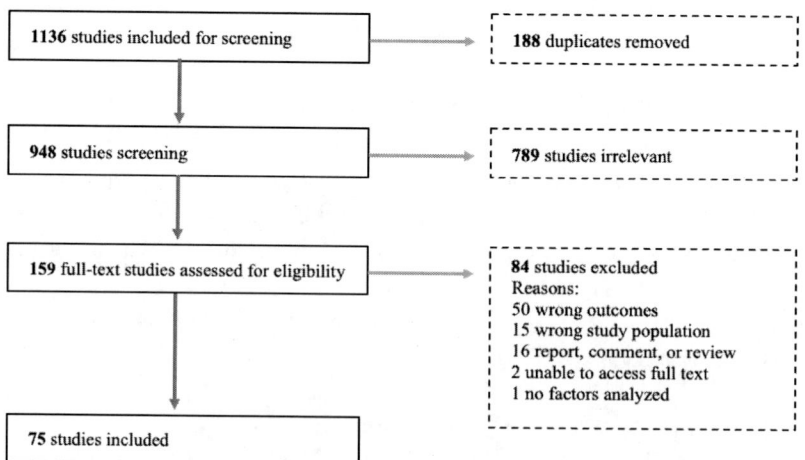

Figure 1. PRISMA diagram summarizing study review process.

Factors influencing inequities in lead exposure in United States children 57

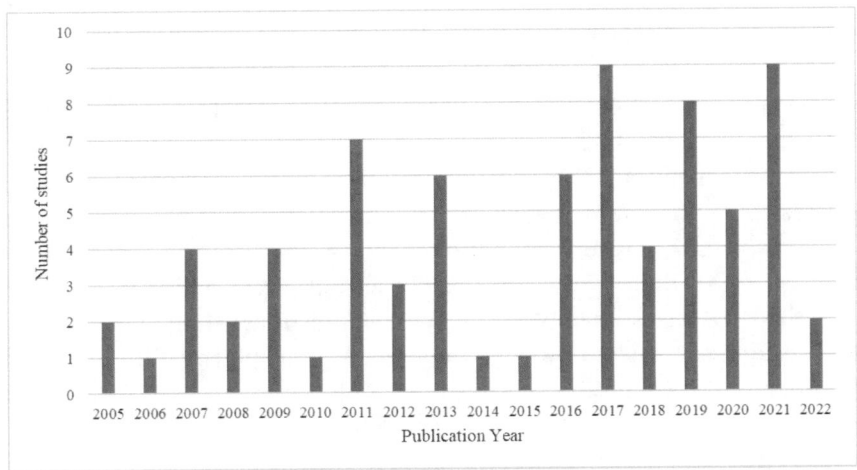

Figure 2. Number of studies by publication year (n = 75).

Although we reviewed only studies published since 2005, some of the studies included analyses of data from earlier time periods (see Figure 3). The earliest year for which BLL data were analyzed was 1976. In a study published in 2021, Egan et al. (16) used nationwide children's BLL data collected as part of the National Health and Nutrition Examination Survey (NHANES) over a 40-year period (1976-2016) to examine changes in population BLLs and in risk factors for elevated BLL over time (16).

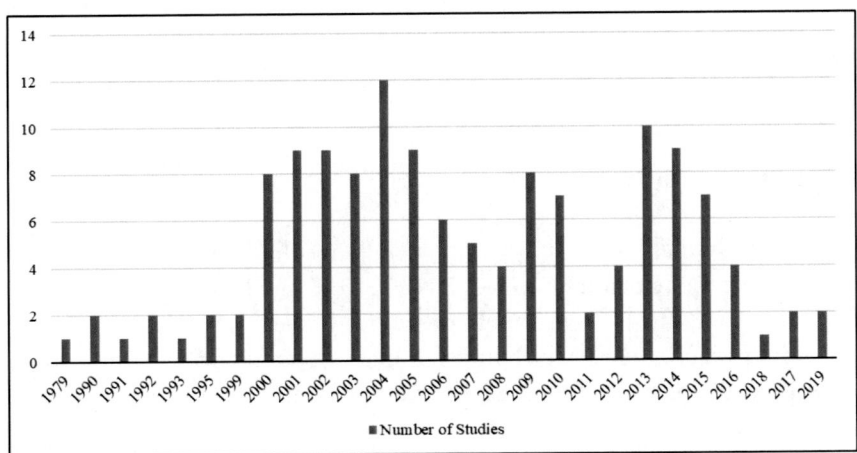

Figure 3. Time periods of data included in studies published since 2005 (n = 133 time points).

Geographic coverage

Of the included studies, 18 analyzed factors and child BLLs from national data including Washington DC. The remaining studies analyzed data from 81 locations representing 27/50 US states and Washington DC, with some studies, 5/75, comparing more than one location (see Figure 4). The two locations with the highest number of studies were New York and Michigan, with 11 and 19 studies, respectively. The lack of recent studies specific to 23 of the 50 US states, mainly in the West but also including some southern, midwestern, and eastern states, is notable given the potential for geographic variation in sources of Pb exposure.

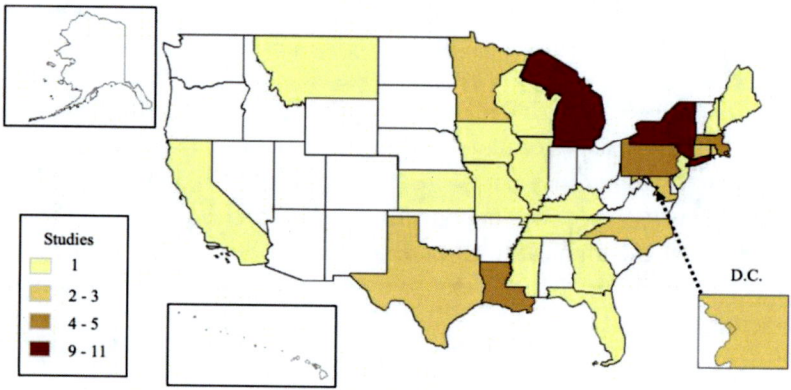

Figure 4. Locations of studies (n = 81 locations).

Age ranges of included children

Among the studies, 70.7% (53/75) included only children ages seven years or less. Among the remaining studies, 20.0% (15/75) included children ages 0 to 18 years, 2.7% (2/75) included children ages 0 to 19 years, and 6.7% (5/75) did not report children's ages but stated that data came from children. While we excluded studies that focused on adult populations, two studies with 19-year-olds were included, because they also covered children under age 19 years (grouping 19 year olds into the 12–19 age range).

Reported blood Pb levels

Central tendency values of BLLs were extracted from 63/75 studies. Children's BLLs ranged between 0 to 164 µg/dL. Measured BLLs declined over time with mean BLLs decreasing by 0.22 µg/dL per year and a median BLLs dropping by 0.18 µg/dL per year from 1979 through 2019 (see Figure 5).

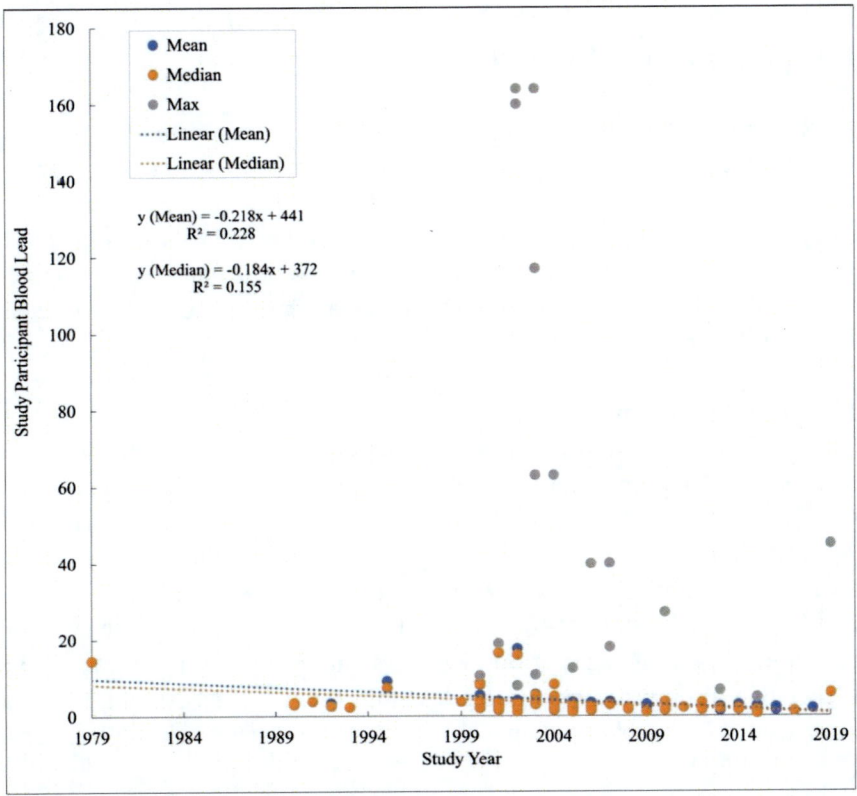

Figure 5. Pooled analysis of blood Pb over time.

The highest values were reported in children living in Michigan (17, 18) including immigrant children and children of immigrants (18), followed by studies that attributed children's exposure to home Pb-based paint hazards in Philadelphia, PA, Cincinnati, OH, and Iowa (19–21), and residential soil Pb concentrations in New Orleans (22). The highest BLL mean was 17.58 µg/dL, reported in a study that evaluated the effect of housing compliance status and time of achieving compliance on BLL changes in 7,377 children ages 0-6 years with BLLs ≥ 10 µg/dL between 1999 and 2004 (21). The highest BLL median was 16.5 µg/dL, which was reported in a study that measured the effectiveness of intense case management to reduce BLLs in exposed children (23). The six studies that compared BLLs by geographic regions reported higher BLLs in northern and midwestern regions (16,24–28). Seasonal variation also was reported, with the highest BLLs occurring during the summer seasons.

Risk factors for children's Pb exposure

A total of 144 factors associated with children's Pb exposure were extracted from the included studies (see Figures 6 and 7). Figure 6 shows the number of studies assessing each factor and whether the studies found that the factor was associated with increased or decreased BLLs for the 77 factors with at least 2 studies. Another 61 factors were analyzed in just one study each; Figure 7 shows effect directions for these factors. Factors were organized into the five levels of the SEM.

Intrapersonal factors

The most frequently assessed intrapersonal factors in order of the number of studies were children's age, sex, race/ethnicity, and place of birth (see Figure 6). In most studies (13/29), male children had higher BLLs than females.

Children under age 5 years had higher BLLs than older children in 37/41 studies. Among newly arrived refugee children, those between the ages of 3 and 7 years had higher BLLs than children < 3 years (29). In New York, children between the ages of 6 to 12 years and living in private housing had higher BLLs compared to children less than 6 years (30). Among Mexican-American children, children up to 12 years of age were at risk of Pb exposure (31).

We also captured BLL differences reported within the 0–5 year age group. In two of 41 studies, children less than one year of age had higher BLLs than children ages two years (19) or 2–3 years (32). In 6 of 38 studies, children less than or equal to two years old had higher BLLs than those aged 3 to 5 years (24, 32–36). In contrast, in four of 38 studies, children aged 2–3 years had the highest BLLs (17, 37–39).

Factors influencing inequities in lead exposure in United States children   61

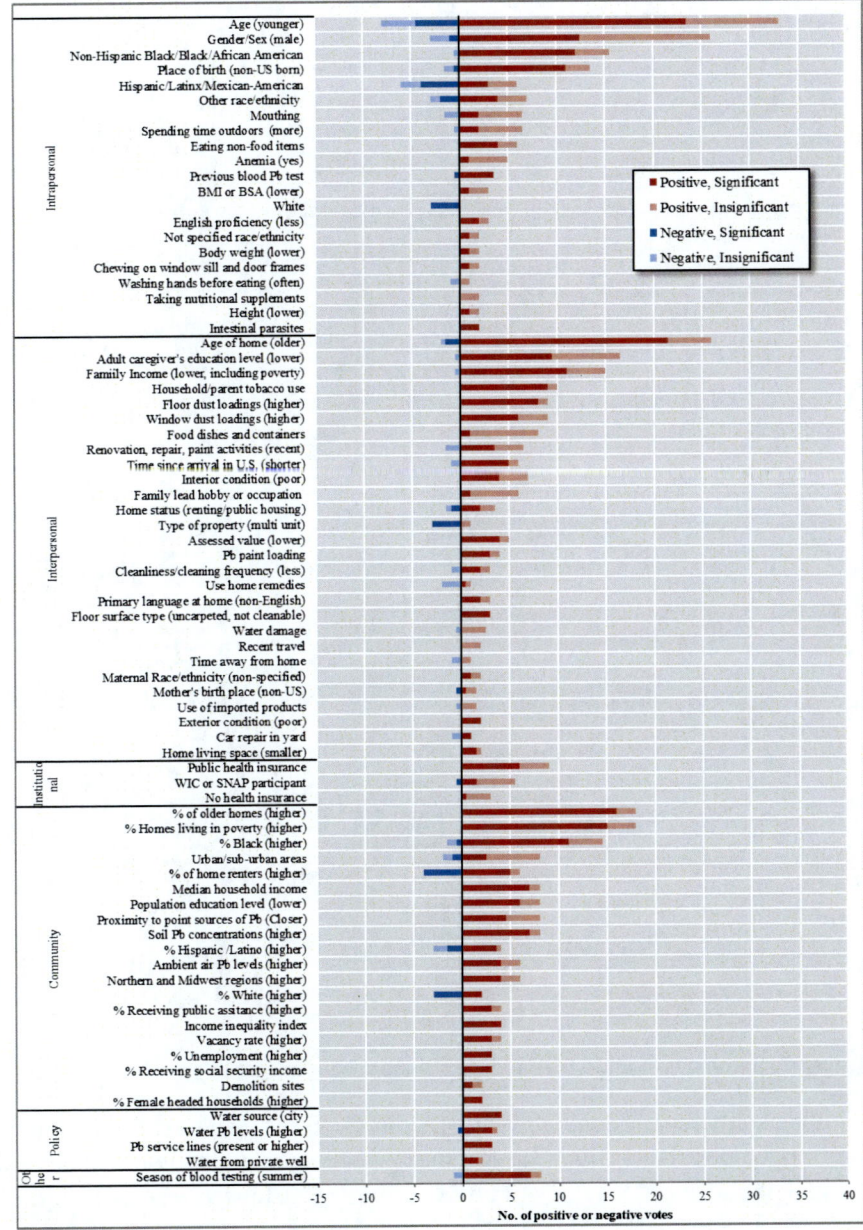

Figure 6. Summary of child blood Pb risk factors with at least two studies (n = 77 factors).

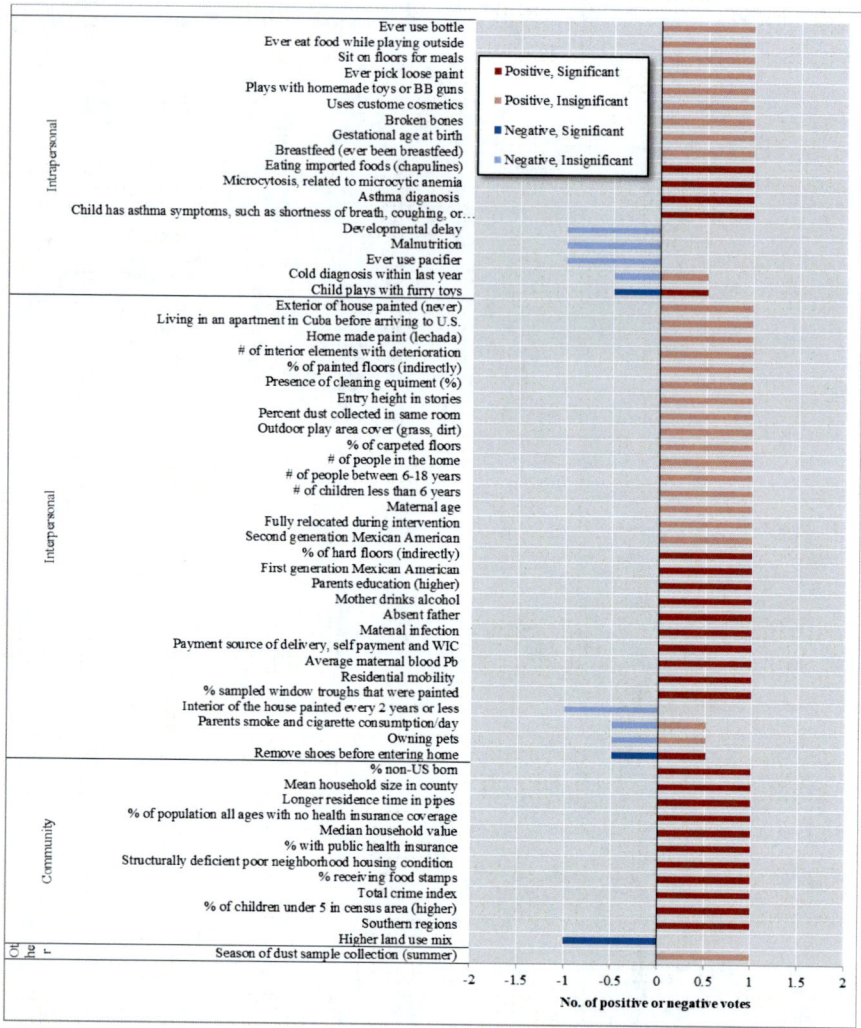

Figure 7. Summary of child blood Pb risk factors with one study (n = 61 factors).

One study reported the highest BLLs in ages less than three years among the refugee population living in Kentucky (40). Another study that analyzed the geographic characteristics of children living in Chicago reported children ages 3 to 4 years had the highest BLLs (41). Among children living in Atlanta metropolitan areas, ages 2 to 5 years had a higher likelihood of having the highest BLLs (42). The differences in BLL by age and study could reflect a combination of spatial variation in Pb exposure sources combined with age-related differences in behaviors, such as mouthing, that affect exposure. For example, an observational study of mouthing behaviors in young children found that children under age two years placed objects in their mouths nearly twice as often as children aged 2–5 years (43).

Apart from age and sex, the intrapersonal factor most often associated with BLLs was race/ethnicity. All 16 studies that examined associations between non-Hispanic Black race and BLL found higher BLLs in this population than among other children, and differences were statistically significant in 12 of the studies. Interestingly, studies of the influence of Hispanic/Mexican-American/Latinx ethnicity on blood Pb had mixed results. In 6/12 studies, Hispanic/Latinx/Mexican-American children had lower BLLs compared to non-Hispanic White children. Perhaps the mixed results may highlight unique and complex interactions among different SEM level factors not yet well understood among Hispanic/Latinx/Mexican-American children. A study by Morales et al. (31) in 2005 attributed variations in reports of associations between Hispanic/Latinx/Mexican-American ethnicity and BLLs to intrapersonal, interpersonal, institutional, and community factors such as gender, age, generational status, home language, family income, education of household, age of housing, and source of drinking water and suggested factors were related to acculturation (31). Among other studies that found a positive and significant association, the increased risk of Pb exposure in Mexican-American children was related to secondhand smoking (44) and ambient air Pb (45). Another key intrapersonal factor associated in most studies (13/15) with increased blood Pb was being born outside of the United States. Children born in Mexico, Africa, West Africa, the Near East, South Asia, Eastern Europe, and the Middle East had higher BLLs than US-born children, on average.

Among the intrapersonal factors related to children's health and development history, having anemia was the most common health condition assessed, evaluated in five studies. Anemia was associated with higher BLL in all but one of the studies (29, 38, 40, 46). It is important to note four of the five studies investigating anemia were based on refugee populations. Having a previous blood test was always positively associated with higher blood Pb whether it was related to a higher initial blood Pb test (2/4 studies, including newborn dried blood spots) (29, 47) or parental report of child testing (37, 48). Histories of lower height, weight, body-mass index (BMI), or body surface area (BSA) were associated with higher blood Pb, but these associations were not always significant.

Among the behaviors that may be related to Pb exposure, spending time outdoors was assessed in the largest number of studies. Only one study found spending time outdoors as a significant factor, while 2/7 studies reported insignificance, 2/7 studies reported mixed findings on significance, and in 2/7 the behavior had no effect. One study found the significance of the behavior was lost when analyzed by race (37).

Mouthing behavior was also assessed in eight studies, with six studies finding positive associations between mouthing and BLLs (though only two reported significant results). Eating non-food items such as paint chips and soil was a strong predictor of blood Pb, with 4/6 studies reporting significance. Washing hands before eating was significantly associated with lower blood Pb in one study (49), and in another study, the behavior did not have an effect (50). Among the factors with one study, eating imported dried grasshoppers (chapulines) was a significant predictor of blood Pb (51), and using costume cosmetics and ever picking loose paint were positively associated (50, 52).

Interpersonal factors
For this analysis, we consider characteristics of the child's family and dwelling as interpersonal factors, consistent with McLeroy's original definition of this level of the SEM. At this level, age of the home was the most frequently studied factor, considered in 28 studies. In 24 studies, BLLs increased with the age of the home. This finding is not surprising, as homes built before the 1978 ban on Pb-based paint have higher probabilities of containing Pb-based paint hazards. Interestingly, one study reported an inverse association between BLLs among Cuban refugees living in Florida and the age of home but later discovered that the new home classification by the city included homes that were built on older structures (before 1979) (53). Another study found that the effect of living in an older home was diminished in the 1 to 5-year children's age group suggesting that for this age group, there are other factors involved (45).

Family income was also commonly considered in studies identified in this review. In 14 studies, family income was inversely related to child blood Pb, such that children from lower-income families (especially families living below the US poverty threshold) were at most risk. Of these, 11 found these associations were significant, while 4 found that blood Pb was positively associated with income, but these results were not statistically significant. Not surprisingly, lower education attainment of the mother, father, or reference adult in the home was also inversely associated with child blood Pb, as this factor is closely associated with family income (54). However, an opposite association was found among South Asian New Yorkers (55).

Another key interpersonal factor associated with increased blood Pb was exposure to tobacco use. Whether exposure was measured by the mother's history of tobacco use, the current family behavior of smoking inside the home, or confirmed secondhand exposure measured in serum cotinine levels in the child, exposure to tobacco use was strongly associated with higher blood Pb. Out of 10 studies that measured tobacco use, 9 found statistically significant associations.

Many studies also evaluated associations between BLLs and Pb in household dust. Floor Pb dust loadings were directly associated with child blood Pb, with 8/9 studies reporting statistically significant associations and 1/9 reporting positive but insignificant associations. Similarly, windowsill Pb dust loadings were directly associated with child blood Pb. In 6/9 studies, associations were significant; in the remaining studies, the association was positive but did not reach significance. Among the studies with positive but insignificant associations, Pb dust loadings from window troughs but not from window sills were significant (56).

While Pb dust loadings generally were significantly associated with higher BLLs, the effects diminished in three studies that conducted further analyses. In one study, the effect of floor and window sill dust Pb loadings went from statistically significant to insignificant after adjusting for the effect of geographic region (24). In another study, the effects of floor and dust Pb loadings were significant on log-transformed child BLLs but insignificant when BLLs were dichotomized into BLL ranges ≥ 5 µg/dL (49). Similarly, in a third study, floor and window Pb dust loadings were significantly associated with overall BLLs but not with BLLs dichotomized into less than 5 µg/dL, 5 to 9 µg/dL, and ≥ 10 µg/dL (57).

Frequent home cleaning was associated with lower blood Pb in one study, as might be expected given that cleaning is expected to decrease dust levels. However, a less clean home was not always associated with children's Pb exposure. In one study, a clean home was negatively but insignificantly associated with higher blood Pb (48).

Deteriorated housing was another risk factor considered in some studies. In 4/7 studies the effect of poor home conditions was significant and in 3/7 the effect was positive but statistically insignificant. Another highly assessed home related condition was home renovation, repair, and paint (RRP) activities. Home RRP activities were associated with increased blood Pb, with the most recent activities (within 12 months) associated with the highest BLLs. The effect was statistically significant in 3/8 and positive but statistically insignificant in 2/8 studies.

Type of property—whether a single-family residence, multi-unit building, or public housing community—was investigated in a few studies. Living in a multi-unit home was associated with lower BLLs compared to single family homes, with 3/4 studies reporting a negative and significant relationship. Living in public housing was negatively associated with child blood Pb, while living in rented homes had mixed effects. The lower risks among residents of public housing and multi-unit structures could reflect beneficial effects of the Lead-Safe Housing Rule, which requires Pb assessment and, where necessary, abatement in housing units receiving federal assistance (58).

Institutional factors

In their foundational paper proposing the SEM framework for health promotion, McLeroy et al. (10) defined institutional factors as "social institutions with organizational characteristics, and formal (and informal) rules and regulations for operation" (10). In this category, we include organizations that provide health insurance, along with local agencies that administer state and federal assistance programs. The latter include the Special Supplemental Nutrition Program for Women, Infants, and Children (WIC) and the Supplemental Nutrition Assistance Program (SNAP). Results on associations between access to health insurance, use of public versus private insurance, and nutrition assistance programs on BLLs is mixed. For example, in an analysis of children born in Pennsylvania in 2015 and 2016 and followed until age two years, Chen et al. (59) found that children whose mothers did not have health insurance at the time of delivery had significantly higher odds of elevated BLLs than children of mothers with Medicaid or with private insurance (59). However, another study found that although children with any insurance had significantly lower BLLs than children without insurance, there was no difference between the two groups in the risk of BLL ≥ 5 µg/dL (38). Similarly, studies including reliance on WIC or SNAP benefits are predictors of BLLs have found mixed results. As an example, the previously mentioned study of the 2015–2016 Pennsylvania birth cohort found significantly lower BLLs in WIC/SNAP participants than in other children (59), but a cross-sectional study of children under age 8 living in Philadelphia neighborhoods with a history of Pb-emitting industry found higher BLLs among children whose families received WIC benefits or food stamps (1). Other studies including WIC/SNAP benefits in predictive models for BLLs were inconclusive (16, 50, 60), finding insignificant or mixed associations between BLLs and use of these benefits.

The inconsistent findings on the effects of health insurance and nutritional benefit programs on BLLs result in part from the high correlation between these variables and socioeconomic status. For example, Wheeler et al. combined health insurance status and reliance on food stamps with multiple measures of household economic status to create a single indicator they called "concentrated disadvantage" (60). This indicator was significantly associated with risks of elevated blood Pb at the Census tract scale. As a result of these correlations, it is difficult to disentangle the effects of these programs on BLLs from the well-established inverse correlation between socioeconomic status and children's BLLs. Nonetheless, health insurance and food assistance programs could provide important opportunities for educational, nutritional, and other interventions to prevent children's Pb exposure or to diminish harm from Pb exposure (e.g., through improved nutrition) since they can serve as conduits to reach at-risk children.

Community factors

The community factors most often considered were measures of socioeconomic status at the neighborhood (e.g., census block or zip code) scale. In 15 of 18 studies, children in areas with a higher percentage of homes living in poverty had significantly higher BLLs than other children, and associations were positive but insignificant in the remaining 3 studies. Several studies also found associations between BLLs and other indicators of overall community socioeconomic status (including median household income, population education levels, and population fraction receiving public assistance). BLLs were consistently higher in socioeconomically disadvantaged communities.

Another commonly assessed community factor was racial composition. Overall, consistent with the intrapersonal effect of Black race on child BLLs, children in areas with higher proportions of Black residents had significantly higher BLLs in most studies including this factor. In three studies, the association was positive and significant when analyzing BLLs as a continuous measure but was negative when analyzing the odds of having BLLs ≥ 5 μg/dL (25, 61) or ≥ 10 μg/dL (62). Similar to the effects of Hispanic ethnicity on child BLLs at the intrapersonal level, areas with higher proportions of Hispanics had mixed associations with BLLs. Nonetheless, of the seven studies that tested associations between neighborhood-scale Hispanic population proportion and BLLs, four found that BLLs were significantly higher in Hispanic than in other neighborhoods.

Another key community factor was the ages of homes in a child's neighborhood. Across 18 studies that included this factor, BLLs were consistently higher in children living in areas with older housing, and associations were statistically significant in the majority (15/18) of studies.

Surprisingly, living in urban/suburban areas rather than in rural areas was not a significant predictor of child Pb exposure in any of the studies. Instead, mixed effects were observed. In 1/10 studies mixed insignificant associations were reported, along with 2/10 studies reporting negative significant and insignificant associations and 5/10 studies reporting positive but insignificant associations.

Community-scale measures of environmental pollution were consistently associated with increased BLLs across studies. In 7/8 studies the association between soil Pb and blood Pb was positive and statistically significant, with soil near the home structure having the largest effect on blood Pb (22, 56). In 1/8 studies, the association was positive but insignificant at two soil Pb thresholds, >150 ppm and < 88 ppm (61). Living near point sources of Pb such as sites registered in the Environmental Protection Agency Toxic Release Inventory, Superfund sites, airports, and transportation corridors was associated with increased BLLs in all eight studies examining this factor, and associations were significant in most of the studies. Ambient air Pb was significantly associated with BLLs in 4/6 studies that analyzed this factor.

Policy factors

The amount of Pb in a child's potable water supply is determined in large part by local, state, and federal policies governing the development, operation, and management of drinking water systems. We identified eight studies that assessed relationships between characteristics of the child's potable water supply and BLLs. All of the studies found significant associations between water supply characteristics and BLLs. However, the measures used to characterize water supplies differed across studies.

Only one study (56) concurrently measured Pb in household tap water and in the blood of resident children. That study followed a cohort of 276 children in Rochester, New York, from age 5–7 months to age 24 months, measuring water Pb, other household Pb exposure sources, and BLLs at various time points. The study found that BLLs were 20.4% higher among those whose water had >5 ppb of Pb, compared to children with lower Pb levels in water.

Other studies used proxies for potential Pb exposure in drinking water. Two studies investigated the effects of the Flint water crisis, in which Pb concentrations spiked after a switch in water source, on children's blood Pb.

One of these, by Sadler et al. (63), used residence time (which is influenced by the distance from the water treatment plant to the child's house) during the crisis as an indicator of Pb exposure; water Pb is expected to be higher at houses that are farther from the treatment plant and are in contact with water mains that may contain Pb for a longer time period. Blood Pb was significantly higher among children in homes where water residence times were longer and also increased more during the water crisis, compared to children in homes with shorter water residence times (63). The second study examined how children's BLLs changed over the course of the water crisis, concluding that BLLs rose by 0.5 µg/dL (on average) during the crisis and that the risks of BLLs ≥ 5 µg/dL increased by a factor of 1.9 to 3.5 depending on neighborhood (64). The Sadler study of the Flint water crisis and one additional study, in Washington, DC (35), investigated whether children's BLLs were associated with the presence of a Pb service line delivering water from the water main to the child's home; both studies found that BLLs were significantly higher among children in homes with Pb service lines.

Three studies assessed associations between BLLs and the type of water source. Two (31,65) were based on data collected as part of the National Health and Nutrition Examination Survey (NHANES); both compared BLLs among children receiving their water from a regulated community water supply to those among children using either bottled water or an unregulated private system (such as a private well). The first study, which used data from 1988-1994 and focused on Mexican-American children, found that children drinking bottled water had significantly lower BLLs than those consuming water from either a community supply or a private well but that there were no significant differences in BLLs between children using the latter two water sources (31). The second study compared NHANES data for all children tested for two time periods, 1988-1994 and 1999-2008 (65). No significant associations between BLLs of children with community water service and those getting their water from private wells were found for the earlier time period; in the later time period, children ages 6-11 years getting their water from a community system had significantly higher BLLs than those using private well water, but associations were not significant for older or younger age groups. More recently, an analysis of blood Pb surveillance data for 59,483 children in Wake County, NC, collected between 2002 and 2017 found that children relying on private well water had significantly higher BLLs and a higher risk of elevated blood Pb than those with community water service. Overall, these studies suggest that Pb in drinking water can contribute significantly to Pb exposure risks.

Discussion

The studies identified in this review reveal that policies implemented over the past 50 years to prevent release of Pb into the environment have yielded tremendous benefits at the population scale but that these benefits have been unequally distributed, with Pb exposure remaining an entrenched problem in some communities. All 13 studies analyzing race at the individual level found that Black children had higher blood Pb concentrations than children of other races. Similarly, a dozen studies published since 2005 have reported higher blood Pb concentrations among children of any race living in majority Black neighborhoods. Children from lower-income families—regardless of race— also remain at significantly higher risk from Pb exposure than children from wealthier families; 14 studies found that blood Pb concentrations increased as family income decreased, and a dozen studies showed higher blood Pb levels in neighborhoods where more families lived in poverty.

Adopting an SEM framework to guide prevention programs could help solve entrenched problems of Pb exposure among low-income and minority children. Figure 8 maps the factors identified in this review on to the SEM framework. This framework illustrates opportunities to intervene at the interpersonal, institutional, community, and policy levels of the SEM. For example, the results suggest that smoking cessation programs for parents and programs to assist families living in older homes with Pb-safe home maintenance and repair could help decrease exposure risks. At the institutional level, given that children without health insurance access have higher blood Pb levels than those with insurance of any kind, programs to expand public insurance to unserved children also could yield benefits. The finding that BLLs are higher among children receiving public insurance than among those with private insurance also suggests the need to strengthen Pb exposure prevention programs for families receiving Medicaid. WIC and SNAP programs also could serve as conduits for reaching at-risk children. Further, enhancements to WIC and SNAP programs to improve access to iron- and calcium-rich foods that prevent Pb uptake could help to decrease Pb exposure risks among low-income children. At the community level, more extensive programs to stabilize Pb-contaminated soils could be developed. At the policy level, continued efforts are needed to decrease risks of exposure to Pb from drinking water, such as through more consistent enforcement of requirements under the Safe Drinking Water Act's Lead and Copper Rule (66) and through policies that extend regulated community water services to areas currently relying on unregulated, private sources.

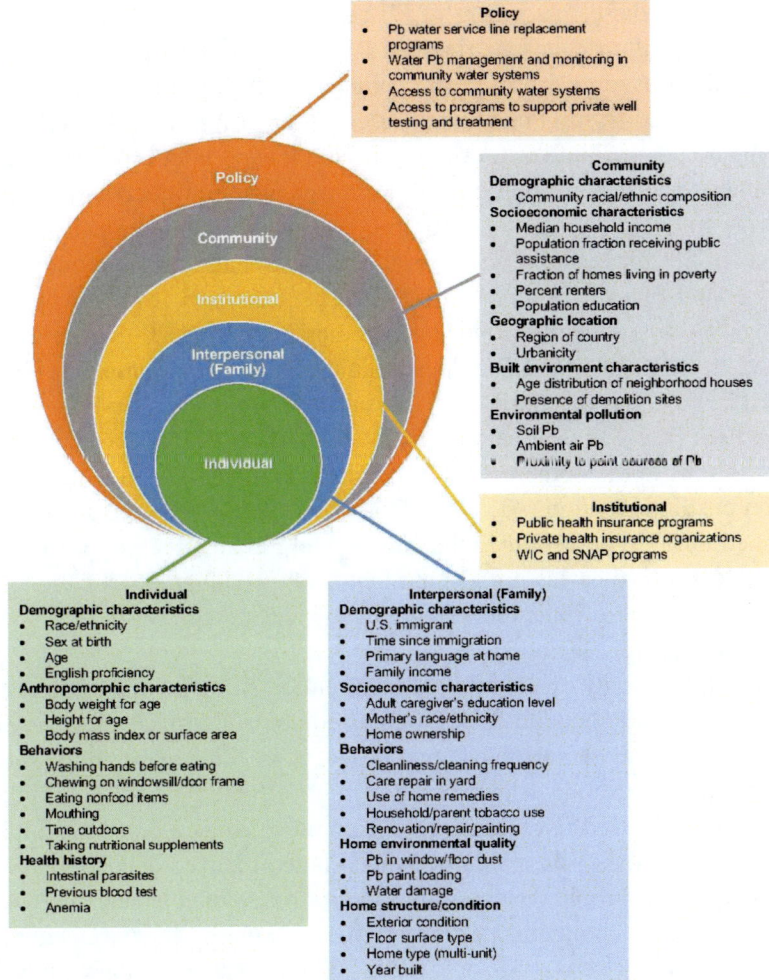

Figure 8. SEM of Pb exposure risk for US children.

Although this review highlights the importance of interventions at all levels of the SEM, the potential effectiveness of specific interventions or packages of interventions, beyond policies already in place, is unknown, because very few recent studies have directly evaluated interventions. Most of the available studies resulted from natural experiments, rather than from pre-planned intervention evaluations (such as randomized-controlled trials). As an example, one study published during the time period covered in this review assessed how the displacement of Pb-contaminated topsoil in New Orleans resulting from hurricanes Katrina and Rita influenced BLLs (79). The study attributed an average 1.65 μg/dL decline in BLLs to the substantial (46%) decrease in median soil Pb occurring after the hurricanes washed away topsoil.

In another example of leveraging a natural experiment, Brown et al. (35) examined the effect on children's BLLs of a change in water disinfectant from chlorine to chloramine in Washington, DC, which unintentionally triggered release of Pb from mineral scale lining the city's water distribution pipes; the study found that the odds of elevated BLLs increased from 1.7 before the change to 3.6 afterwards (35). Many studies pre-dating 2005 also leveraged natural experiments, for example examining how population blood Pb levels tracked with changes in airborne Pb resulting from the ban on Pb in gasoline (69). Clark et al. (48) studied the effects of HUD-supported Pb hazard control interventions in the homes of 1,273 children on their BLLs over a three-year period post intervention (48). They found that BLLs of participating children declined by 37% on average by year two and remained steady through year three. However, this was not a controlled study. HUD grantees were allowed to choose their own intervention strategies, and no control houses (without interventions) were included.

We located only one controlled intervention study published since 2005. Brown et al. (23) conducted a randomized-controlled trial of an intensive home visiting and parental education program, in comparison to the standard of care, among Rhode Island children with elevated BLLs (23). Program participants received five home visits from nurses over a one-year follow-up period. During the visits, parents received individualized education about Pb hazards, and household dust and soil samples were collected and analyzed for Pb, with results communicated to parents as soon as they were available. Control families received one or two educational visits by an outreach worker, who delivered standardized (not customized) educational materials, and no samples were collected. The study found that the intervention significantly decreased Pb in household dust, but there was no effect on BLLs. The many opportunities for intervention suggested by the SEM, plus the paucity of well-controlled studies of interventions, suggest the need for further study to identify the intervention approaches most likely to succeed in reaching at-risk children.

Improved risk assessment methods to identify children most likely to have higher BLLs also are needed. To identify areas where children are most at risk, state health departments typically use binary or categorical indicators of Pb exposure potential, typically at the zip code scale, based on age of housing and percentage of homes in poverty (17). However, these indicators have a very low correlation with measured BLLs; Kaplowitz et al. (17) found that a binary indicator based on zip code explained only 7.6% of the variance in measured BLLs among children tested in Michigan. Recent initiatives under way by CDC and others are seeking to develop more accurate risk screening methods, but these are not yet used in practice (70). In addition, routine screening typically is recommended only for children under age 6 years, but this review indicates that in some cases, children in older age groups can have higher BLLs.

Limitations

There are several limitations in our review. One limitation is related to the search and eligibility criteria for including articles. Factors identified may have been incomplete due to limitations of the search terms, potentially excluding articles that may have been relevant but lacked our keywords in the title and abstract. Also, our search was limited to what PubMed identified, possibly excluding articles that can be found through other scientific libraries such as Google Scholar and EBSCO. Another limitation is that our review did not go into more depth to analyze the effects of the interactions of the risk factors identified in our review. While interactions between risk factors are important to include in SEMs, we were constricted by time and resources to extend our review to understand and extract interactions. Lastly, another limitation is related bias. While our team followed PRISMA guidelines for research reviews, there is a possibility that information extracted from articles could have been evaluated differently based on each reviewer's subjective decisions and biases.

Conclusion

Childhood Pb poisoning is an old problem that needs new approaches to eradicate its long-lasting effects. The proposed SEM is a step closer to understanding and addressing the Pb exposure inequities that children in the US experience and a step closer to informing equitable primary intervention strategies.

Acknowledgments

We would like to recognize and thank Aralia Pawlick, Lauren Kwan, and Alyson Alde for contributing to the reviewing process of the studies. We also want to express gratitude to the Break the Cycle of Children's Environmental Health Disparities program by Break the Cycle of Health Disparities Inc and the Southeast Pediatric Environmental Health Specialty Unit (PEHSU) at Emory University, as well as the participating mentors and mentees for their guidance and feedback on this study. Special recognition to Jaqueline MacDonald Gibson for her mentorship and support in participating in the program.

References

[1] Dignam T, Kaufmann RB, LeStourgeon L, Brown MJ. Control of lead sources in the United States, 1970-2017: Public health progress and current challenges to eliminating lead exposure. J Public Health Manag Pract 2019;25(Suppl 1):S13–22.
[2] McFarland MJ, Hauer ME, Reuben A. Half of US population exposed to adverse lead levels in early childhood. Proc Natl Acad Sci 2022;119 (11):e2118631119.
[3] Center for Disease Control and Prevention. Health effects of lead exposure. Atlanta, GA: CDC, 2022. URL: https://www.cdc.gov/nceh/lead/prevention/health-effects.htm.
[4] Bellinger DC. Neurological and behavioral consequences of childhood lead exposure. PLoS Med 2008;5(5):e115.
[5] Bellinger DC. Very low lead exposures and children's neurodevelopment. Curr Opin Pediatr 2008;20(2):172–7.
[6] Lanphear BP, Hornung R, Khoury J, Yolton K, Baghurst P, Bellinger DC, et al. Low-Level Environmental Lead Exposure and Children's Intellectual Function: An International Pooled Analysis. Environ Health Perspect. 2005 Jul;113(7):894–9.
[7] Canfield RL, Henderson CR, Cory-Slechta DA, Cox C, Jusko TA, Lanphear BP. Intellectual Impairment in children with blood lead concentrations below 10 μg per deciliter. N Engl J Med 2003;348(16):1517–26.
[8] Del Rio M, Sobin C, Hettiarachchi G. Biological factors that impact variability of lead absorption and BLL estimation in children: Implications for child blood lead level testing practices. J Environ Health 2022;85(5):18-26.
[9] Mielke HW, Zahran S. The urban rise and fall of air lead (Pb) and the latent surge and retreat of societal violence. Environ Int 2012;43:48–55.
[10] McLeroy KR, Bibeau D, Stecker A, Glanz K. An ecological perspective on health promotion programs. Health Educ Quart 2016;15(4). URL: https://journals.sagepub.com/doi/10.1177/109019818801500401.

[11] Page MJ, McKenzie JE, Bossuyt PM, Boutron I, Hoffmann TC, Mulrow CD, et al. The PRISMA 2020 statement: An updated guideline for reporting systematic reviews. BMJ 2021 Mar 29:n71.
[12] PRISMA. URL: http://www.prisma-statement.org/.
[13] Covidence. Better systematic review management. URL: https://www.covidence.org/.
[14] Flodgren G, Eccles MP, Shepperd S, Scott A, Parmelli E, Beyer FR. An overview of reviews evaluating the effectiveness of financial incentives in changing healthcare professional behaviours and patient outcomes. Cochrane Database Syst Rev 2011;2011(7):CD009255.
[15] George AN, Stewart JR, Evans JC, Gibson JM. Risk of antibiotic-resistant staphylococcus aureus dispersion from hog farms: A critical review. Risk Anal 2020;40(8):1645–65.
[16] Egan KB, Cornwell CR, Courtney JG, Ettinger AS. Blood lead levels in US children ages 1–11 Years, 1976–2016. Environ Health Perspect 2021;129(3):037003.
[17] Kaplowitz SA, Perlstadt H, Post LA. Comparing lead poisoning risk assessment methods: census block group characteristics vs. zip codes as predictors. Public Health Rep 2010;125(2):234–45.
[18] Kaplowitz SA, Perlstadt H, Dziura JD, Post LA. Behavioral and environmental explanations of elevated blood lead levels in immigrant children and children of immigrants. J Immigr Minor Health 2016;18(5):979–86.
[19] Braun JM, Yolton K, Newman N, Jacobs DE, Taylor M, Lanphear BP. Residential dust lead levels and the risk of childhood lead poisoning in United States children. Pediatr Res 2021;90(4):896–902.
[20] Carrel M, Zahrieh D, Young SG, Oleson J, Ryckman KK, Wels B, et al. High prevalence of elevated blood lead levels in both rural and urban Iowa newborns: Spatial patterns and area-level covariates. PLoS One 2017;12(5):e0177930.
[21] Rappazzo K, Cummings CE, Himmelsbach RM, Tobin R. The effect of housing compliance status on children's blood lead levels. Arch Env Occup Health 2007;62(2):81–5.
[22] Mielke HW, Gonzales CR, Powell ET, Mielke PW. Environmental and health disparities in residential communities of New Orleans: the need for soil lead intervention to advance primary prevention. Env Int 2013;51:73–81.
[23] Brown MJ, McLaine P, Dixon S, Simon P. A randomized, community-based trial of home visiting to reduce blood lead levels in children. Pediatrics 2006;117(1):147–53.
[24] Scott LL, Nguyen LM. Geographic region of residence and blood lead levels in US children: results of the National Health and Nutrition Examination Survey. Int Arch Occup Env Health 2011;84(5):513–22.
[25] Hauptman M, Niles JK, Gudin J, Kaufman HW. Individual- and community-level factors associated with detectable and elevated blood lead levels in US children: Results from a national clinical laboratory. JAMA Pediatr 2021;175(12):1252–60.

[26] Keller B, Faciano A, Tsega A, Ehrlich J. Epidemiologic characteristics of children with blood lead levels ≥45 µg/dL. J Pediatr 2017;180:229–34.

[27] McClure LF, Niles JK, Kaufman HW. Blood lead levels in young children: US, 2009-2015. J Pediatr 2016;175:173–81.

[28] Benson SM, Talbott EO, Brink LL, Wu C, Sharma RK, Marsh GM. Environmental lead and childhood blood lead levels in US children: NHANES, 1999-2006. Arch Env Occup Health 2017;72(2):70–8.

[29] Eisenberg KW, van Wijngaarden E, Fisher SG, Korfmacher KS, Campbell JR, Fernandez ID, et al. Blood lead levels of refugee children resettled in Massachusetts, 2000 to 2007. Am J Public Health 2011;101(1):48–54.

[30] Chiofalo JM, Golub M, Crump C, Calman N. Pediatric blood lead levels within New York City public versus private housing, 2003-2017. Am J Public Health 2019;109(6):906–11.

[31] Moralez LS, Gutierrez P, Escarce JJ. Demographic and socioeconomic factors associated with blood lead levels among Mexican-American children and adolescents in the United States. Public Health Rep 2005;120(4):448–54.

[32] Ford DM, Margaritis V, Mendelsohn AB. Characteristics of childhood lead poisoning among Tennessee children ages one to five years, 2009-2013. Public Health 2016;136:188–91.

[33] Teye SO, Yanosky JD, Cuffee Y, Weng X, Luquis R, Farace E, et al. Exploring persistent racial/ethnic disparities in lead exposure among American children aged 1-5 years: results from NHANES 1999-2016. Int Arch Occup Env Health 2021;94(4):723–30.

[34] Jones RL, Homa DM, Meyer PA, Brody DJ, Caldwell KL, Pirkle JL, et al. Trends in blood lead levels and blood lead testing among US children aged 1 to 5 years, 1988-2004. Pediatrics 2009;123(3):e376-85.

[35] Brown MJ, Raymond J, Homa D, Kennedy C, Sinks T. Association between children's blood lead levels, lead service lines, and water disinfection, Washington, DC, 1998-2006. Env Res 2011;111(1):67–74.

[36] Gleason K, Shine JP, Shobnam N, Rokoff LB, Suchanda HS, Ibne Hasan MOS, et al. Contaminated turmeric is a potential source of lead exposure for children in rural Bangladesh. J Environ Public Health 2014;2014:730636.

[37] Nriagu J, Senthamarai-Kannan R, Jamil H, Fakhori M, Korponic S. Lead poisoning among Arab American and African American children in the Detroit metropolitan area, Michigan. Bull Environ Contam Toxicol 2011;87(3):238–44.

[38] Yeter D, Banks EC, Aschner M. Disparity in risk factor severity for early childhood blood lead among predominantly African-American Black children: The 1999 to 2010 US NHANES. Int J Env Res Public Health 2020;17(5).

[39] Gibson JM, Fisher M, Clonch A, MacDonald JM, Cook PJ. Children drinking private well water have higher blood lead than those with city water. Proc Natl Acad Sci 2020;117(29):16898–907.

[40] Kotey S, Carrico R, Wiemken TL, Furmanek S, Bosson R, Nyantakyi F, et al. Elevated blood lead levels by length of time from resettlement to health screening in Kentucky refugee children. Am J Public Health 2018;108(2):270–6.

[41] Oyana TJ, Margai FM. Geographic analysis of health risks of pediatric lead exposure: A golden opportunity to promote healthy neighborhoods. Arch Env Occup Health 2007;62(2):93–104.

[42] Dickinson-Copeland CM, Immergluck LC, Britez M, Yan F, Geng R, Edelson M, et al. Increased risk of sub-clinical blood lead levels in the 20-County Metro Atlanta, Georgia Area—A laboratory surveillance-based study. Int J Environ Res Public Health 2021;18(10):5163.

[43] Tulve NS, Suggs JC, Mccurdy T, Cohen Hubal EA, Moya J. Frequency of mouthing behavior in young children. J Expo Sci Environ Epidemiol 2002;12 (4):259–64.

[44] Richter PA, Bishop EE, Wang J, Kaufmann R. Trends in tobacco smoke exposure and blood lead levels among youths and adults in the United States: The National Health and Nutrition Examination Survey, 1999-2008. Prev Chronic Dis 2013;10:E213.

[45] Richmond-Bryant J, Meng Q, Cohen J, Davis JA, Svendsgaard D, Brown JS, et al. Effect measure modification of blood lead–air lead slope factors. J Expo Sci Environ Epidemiol 2015;25(4):411–6.

[46] Seifu S, Tanabe K, Hauck FR. The prevalence of elevated blood lead levels in foreign-born refugee children upon arrival to the US and the adequacy of follow-up treatment. J Immigr Minor Health 2020;22(1):10–6.

[47] Archer NP, Bradford CM, Klein DM, Barnes J, Smith LJ, Villanacci JF. Relationship between prenatal lead exposure and infant blood lead levels. Matern Child Health J 2012;16(7):1518–24.

[48] Clark S, Galke W, Succop P, Grote J, McLaine P, Wilson J, et al. Effects of HUD-supported lead hazard control interventions in housing on children's blood lead. Environ Res 2011;111(2):301–11.

[49] Dignam T, Pomales A, Werner L, Newbern EC, Hodge J, Nielsen J, et al. Assessment of child lead exposure in a Philadelphia community, 2014. J Public Health Manag Pract 2019;25(1):53–61.

[50] Plotinsky RN, Straetemans M, Wong LY, Brown MJ, Dignam T, Dana Flanders W, et al. Risk factors for elevated blood lead levels among African refugee children in New Hampshire, 2004. Environ Res 2008;108(3):404–12.

[51] Handley MA, Hall C, Sanford E, Diaz E, Gonzalez-Mendez E, Drace K, et al. Globalization, binational communities, and imported food risks: results of an outbreak investigation of lead poisoning in Monterey County, California. Am J Public Health 2007;97(5):900–6.

[52] Perez AL, Nembhard M, Monnot A, Bator D, Madonick E, Gaffney SH. Child and adult exposure and health risk evaluation following the use of metal- and metalloid-containing costume cosmetics sold in the United States. Regul Toxicol Pharmacol 2017;84:54–63.

[53] Trepka MJ, Pekovic V, Santana JC, Zhang G. Risk factors for lead poisoning among Cuban refugee children. Public Health Rep 2005;120(2):179–85.

[54] Parents' low education leads to low income, despite full-time employment. NCCP. URL: https://www.nccp.org/publication/parents-low-education-leads-to-low-income-despite-full-time-employment/.

[55] Hore P, Ahmed MS, Sedlar S, Saper RB, Nagin D, Clark N. Blood lead levels and potential risk factors for lead exposures among South Asians in New York City. J Immigr Minor Health 2017;19(6):1322–9.

[56] Spanier AJ, Wilson S, Ho M, Hornung R, Lanphear BP. The contribution of housing renovation to children's blood lead levels: A cohort study. Environ Health 2013;12:72.

[57] Cluett R, Fleisch A, Decker K, Frohmberg E, Smith AE. Findings of a statewide environmental lead inspection program targeting homes of children with blood Lead levels as low as 5 μg/dL. J Public Health Manag Pract 2019;25(Suppl 1):S76–83.

[58] Information and guidance for HUD's lead safe housing rule. URL: https://www.hud.gov/program_offices/healthy_homes/enforcement/lshr.

[59] Chen YH, Ma ZQ, Watkins SM. Effects of individual and neighborhood characteristics on childhood blood lead testing and elevated blood lead levels, A Pennsylvania Birth Cohort analysis. J Prim Care Commun Health 2021;12:21501327211017780.

[60] Wheeler DC, Boyle J, Raman S, Nelson EJ. Modeling elevated blood lead level risk across the United States. Sci Total Environ 2021;769:145237.

[61] Pavilonis B, Cheng Z, Johnson G, Maroko A. Lead, soils, and children: An ecological analysis of lead contamination in parks and elevated blood lead levels in Brooklyn, New York. Arch Env Contam Toxicol 2022;82(1):1–10.

[62] Brink LL, Talbott EO, Sharma RK, Marsh GM, Wu WC, Rager JR, et al. Do US ambient air lead levels have a significant impact on childhood blood lead levels: results of a national study. J Environ Public Health 2013;2013:278042.

[63] Sadler RC, LaChance J, Hanna-Attisha M. Social and built environmental correlates of predicted blood lead levels in the Flint Water Crisis. Am J Public Health 2017;107(5):763–9.

[64] Zahran S, McElmurry SP, Sadler RC. Four phases of the Flint Water Crisis: Evidence from blood lead levels in children. Environ Res 2017;157:160–72.

[65] Richmond-Bryant J, Meng Q, Davis JA, Cohen J, Svendsgaard D, Brown JS, et al. A multi-level model of blood lead as a function of air lead. Sci Total Environ 2013;461–462:207–13.

[66] US Environmental Protection Agency. Lead and copper rule, 2015. URL: https://www.epa.gov/dwreginfo/lead-and-copper-rule.

[67] Mielke HW, Gonzales CR, Powell ET. Soil lead and children's blood lead disparities in pre- and post-hurricane Katrina New Orleans (USA). Int J Environ Res Public Health 2017;14(4):407.

[68] Mielke HW, Gonzales CR, Powell ET, Laidlaw MAS, Berry KJ, Mielke PW Jr, et al. The concurrent decline of soil lead and children's blood lead in New Orleans. Proc Natl Acad Sci USA 2019;116(44):22058–64.

[69] The relationship between gasoline lead and blood lead in the United States. URL: https://www.scb.se/contentassets/ca21efb41fee47d293bbee5bf7be7fb3/the-relationship-between-gasoline-lead-and-blood-lead-in-the-united-states.pdf.

[70] Lead data mapping to prioritize US locations for whole-of-government exposure prevention efforts: State of the science, federal collaborations, and remaining challenges. AJPH 2022;112(S7). URL: https://ajph.aphapublications.org/doi/full/10.2105/AJPH.2022.307051.

Submitted: November 19, 2022. *Revised:* December 12, 2022. *Accepted:* January 03, 2023.

Chapter 5

Characterizing lead exposure in households that depend on private wells for drinking water

Alyson Alde[1], MS
Frank Stillo[2], PhD
Abhishek Komandur[3], MSPH
James Harrington[4], PhD
and Jacqueline MacDonald Gibson[5,*], PhD

[1]Department of Environmental and Occupational Health, School of Public Health, Indiana University, Bloomington, Indiana, United States of America
[2]Geosyntec Consultants, Raleigh, North Carolina, United States of America
[3]Department of Environmental Sciences and Engineering, Gillings School of Global Public Health, University of North Carolina, Chapel Hill, North Carolina, United States of America
[4]RTI International, Research Triangle Park, North Carolina, United States of America
[5]Department of Civil, Construction, and Environmental Engineering, North Carolina State University, Raleigh, North Carolina, United States of America

Abstract

Evidence accumulated over the past several decades indicates there is no safe level of exposure to lead. Although the Safe Drinking Water Act limits exposure to lead from municipal water supplies, no such protection exists for private wells. Research suggests United States children relying on private wells have increased risk from lead exposure compared to

---

* **Correspondence:** Jacqueline MacDonald Gibson, PhD, Head, Department of Civil, Construction, and Environmental Engineering, North Carolina State University, Raleigh, North Carolina, United States. Email: jmacdon@ncsu.edu.

In: Environmental Health Disparities
Editors: I. Leslie Rubin and Joav Merrick
ISBN: 979-8-89113-487-4
© 2024 Nova Science Publishers, Inc.

those served by a regulated water system. However, no prior US studies have concurrently measured water and blood lead levels in homes using private wells. To assess these associations, we collected blood, tap water and household dust samples from 89 participants using private wells for drinking water. A multivariable regression was performed to examine the association between well water lead and blood lead, controlling for lead in dust and other confounders. Although water and blood lead levels were not directly associated, filtering water was associated with a 32% decrease in blood lead ($p < 0.05$). Additionally, using a filter was significantly associated with decreased risk high lead in water ($p = 0.01$). We found significant racial disparities in access to water filters. Among African American or Native American participants, 38% had a water filter, compared to 83% of other participants ($p < 0.001$). This study highlights that drinking unfiltered private well water may increase the risk of exposure to lead and that racial disparities in access to and use of water filters in homes relying on private wells, may therefore contribute to longstanding disparities in children's blood lead.

Introduction

Lead is a neurotoxicant that has been proven to have no safe level of exposure (1). Once ingested or inhaled, it can cross the blood-brain barrier, where it can interfere with normal brain development and function. Because children's organs are still developing, they are most vulnerable to lead's neurotoxic effects (2). Additionally, due to behavioral characteristics and metabolism, children are at a greatest risk for lead exposure and absorption (2). Many studies over the last several decades have linked early-life lead exposure to decreased academic achievement (3), attention-related behaviors (4) and problematic behaviors at home and school (4). Additionally, these effects can carry into adulthood (5). Evidence also is mounting that lead exposure poses health risks in adults (1, 6–9). Multiple studies have found associations between chronic lead exposure and increased risk of heart disease, kidney disease and high blood pressure (1, 7–9). Currently, research is exploring an association between lead exposure and degenerative diseases such as cataracts and dementia (8). Some studies suggest there may be a causal relationship between chronic lead exposure in adulthood and accelerated cognitive decline (6). Furthermore, research suggests that pregnant people exposed to lead are at a higher risk for infertility, miscarriage, still birth, premature birth, and low birthweight (7). Although a causal relationship has yet to be defined, research is exploring the association between lead exposure and several types of cancers (7). Additionally, community surveys have found an association between increased mortality and lead exposure (8).

At the population level, blood lead levels have decreased significantly over time in the United States (US). For example, in 2018, the US Centers for Disease Control and Prevention (CDC) reported that an estimated 2.6% of US children under age six years had a blood lead level (BLL) at or above 5 µg/dL—half the prevalence reported in 2012 (10). This decrease reflects several decades of national legislation to limit the use of lead in industrial and consumer products (11). Lead-based paint was banned in 1978 (11), and leaded gasoline was officially phased out in 1996 (12). The Safe Drinking Water Act was introduced in 1974, but it did not include lead exposure prevention policy until 1986 (13). In 1986, Congress prohibited the use of pipes, fittings, solder, and flux that were not "lead free." In this amendment, "lead free" allowed solder and flux to contain up to 0.2% lead and pipes to contain to contain up to 8% lead (14). In 2011, the Reduction of Lead in Drinking Water Act was passed (14). This act adjusted the definition of "lead free" by reducing the weighted average of lead in all wetted plumbing structures to not exceed 0.25% of the total weight of the plumbing features (14).

Although US blood lead levels have declined, exposure to environmental lead remains a public health issue. As a response to growing evidence of lead's neurotoxic effects in even the smallest doses, in November 2021 the CDC adjusted the reference level for elevated blood lead from 5 µg/dL to 3.5 µg/dL (10). An estimated 600,000 US children have blood lead levels above this new threshold (15). Non-Hispanic black children continue to have higher blood lead levels than their white counterparts. A 2021 study of approximately 7,000 children nationwide during 2013–2016, found that non-Hispanic black children were 50% more likely to have elevated blood lead than non-Hispanic white children (16). Given the well-established neurocognitive and other damaging effects of lead, longstanding disparities in exposure may contribute to disparities in children's health and development.

One important persistant source of environmental lead exposure is drinking water. Lead contamination of water usually occurs from the dissolution of lead from pipes and fixtures (15). To prevent lead contamination through this route, municipal water systems monitor and control the corrosivity of the water they distribute (15). This lead prevention strategy gained public attention during the Flint, Michigan, water crisis, which was caused by failures in the city's corrosion control program (17). When the city transitioned from sourcing their water supply from the Detroit Water and

Sewerage Department, they used the Flint River as their temporary water source (18). Because the city did not take the proper precautions to control the water's corrosivity, lead was released from lead-bearing water service lines and household plumbing and fixtures and, as a result, tens of thousands of families were exposed to lead from their drinking water (18).

The Flint water crisis resulted from the failure to comply with legally mandated requirements for water monitoring and treatment that community water systems must follow under the Safe Drinking Water Act. These requirements do not apply to the 13% of Americans who rely on private wells (19). The lack of routine monitoring and treatment may leave these consumers at risk from lead in their drinking water. The US Environmental Protection Agency (EPA) recognizes a drinking water system as "public" when it has at least 15 service connections or when it provides drinking water for at least 25 people for at least 60 days a year (20). Because private wells do not meet these thresholds, households relying on private wells are fully responsible for monitoring and treating their drinking water.

A few states require testing of well water for lead upon initial construction of the well and/or when property is transferred, however, no state requires routine testing (21). Multiple studies have shown that households relying on private well water generally do not test their water quality on a regular basis, if ever (22). This lack of testing is alarming because recent studies in multiple US communities have found elevated concentrations of lead in private well water (22–27). These studies suggest that children relying on a private well for their drinking water may be at increased risk for lead exposure, compared to those in homes served by a community water system.

In some parts of the country, there are racial disparities in access to a regulated community water supply, with ethnic minority groups having to rely on private wells even though they are in close proximity to nearby community water systems (28–31). For example, a study in Wake County, North Carolina, found that as the population of Black residents in areas adjacent to cities and towns increased, so did the odds of lacking a connection to a community water supply and having to rely on a private well (32). Racial disparities in access to municipal drinking water also has been reported in multiple other states, including California (28, 29), Texas (30), Florida (31), and Ohio (29). It is possible that in such areas, exclusion from community water service could contribute to observed disparities in children's blood lead levels.

Despite the potential risks from lead exposure, limited research has been done to examine blood lead levels in children or adults who get their drinking water from private wells. A 2020 study in Wake County, NC, reported that children in households relying on private well had a 25% increased risk of elevated blood lead levels when compared to children served by a municipal water utility that practices corrosion control (33). This study matched data about household water sources in the county to blood lead surveillance data but did not collect concurrent measurements of lead in blood and lead in water, limiting the ability to draw causal conclusions. The gap in knowledge about the impacts of lead in private well water on blood lead may contribute to the lack of awareness of this potential risk, which in turn could increase the risk of lead exposure for the millions of families relying on private well water.

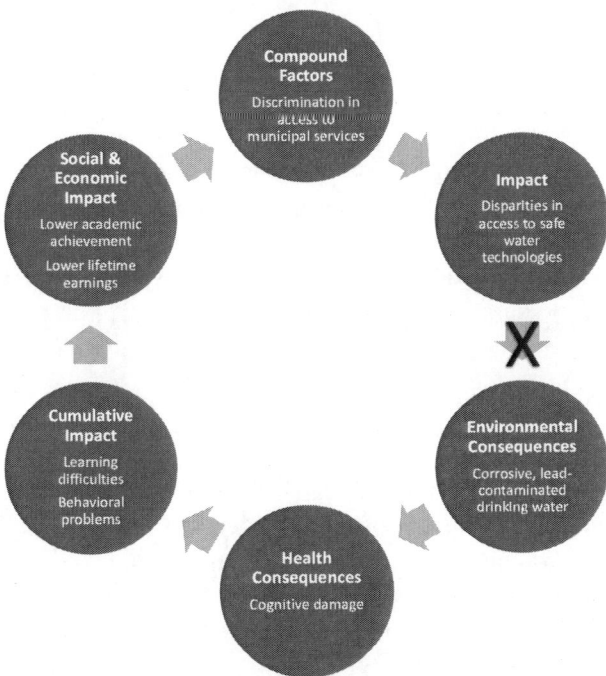

Figure 1. The cycle of childhood environmental health disparities pertaining to lead exposure via unregulated drinking water.

Since limited research has been conducted to fully examine risks of exposure to lead in private well water, this project acts as a first step to assess the magnitude of this risk to inform intervention strategies. Considering the irreversible cognitive deficits lead exposure can inflict on children, the inequitable access to safe drinking water may be an important contributor to disparities in children's health and development that may last a lifetime. This project's goal is to gain a better understanding of lead exposure of populations relying on private wells so that critical interventions—such a well water stewardship education, low-cost filters, financial support to maintain the filters, and in some cases development of community water supplies—may be implemented to eliminate lead exposure completely. This project seeks to break the cycle of environmental health disparities by examining whether access to safe water technologies is associated with exposure to lead in drinking water (see Figure 1).

Our study

To characterize blood lead levels in people who get their drinking water from private wells, this study used a cross-sectional design. We recruited 89 participants in North Carolina who rely on private wells for drinking water to test household tap water and participants' blood samples for lead. Dust samples were also collected as controls to represent other potential routes of exposure (paint and dust). A household questionnaire was conducted to understand household and behavioral characteristics. This study was approved by the Indiana University IRB # 2003976342.

Sample population and recruitment

Participants were eligible for this study if they 1) lived in a household that obtained their primary source of drinking water from a private well and 2) lived in North Carolina. To identify eligible participants, we used a variety of recruitment strategies. We partnered with several community organizations – American Indian Mothers, Robeson County Department of Health, and the Robeson County Special Supplemental Nutrition Program for Women, Infants, and Children (WIC) office. These organizations helped us identify eligible households, posted flyers in their offices and on their social media pages, and mailed flyers to their organization's members and participants. Additionally, we mailed letters to households from lists of private well owners developed in our prior research (34, 35), relied on word-of-mouth strategies from current and previous participants, went door-to-door, and created a website for potential participants to visit and sign up. All participants received a $75 Visa gift card. Participants who recruited a household received an additional $25 visa gift card.

Sample collection

To characterize the relationship between blood lead levels and drinking water sourced from a private well, three types of samples were collected: water, dust, and blood. In addition, a household questionnaire was conducted to determine characteristics of the home and well, demographic information, and behaviors of participants that might be associated with lead exposure. The research team went to the homes of the participants for sample collection and survey administration.

Blood sample collection and analysis

For 59 participants, blood samples were collected by a trained phlebotomist during the initial visit. The phlebotomist collected two five mL samples from the antecubital region using 6.0 mL vacutainer K2 EDTA 10.8 mg tubes. After collection, tubes were stored in a refrigerator until ready for analysis. All samples were analyzed within 30 days of collection. Lead and other toxic heavy metals were analyzed at RTI International laboratories via inductively coupled plasms mass spectrometry (ICPMS) using RTI's published laboratory procedures (36).

Due to barriers from the hesitation of participants to participate in a venous blood draw, the research team transitioned to a capillary sample partway through the study, collecting capillary samples for 30 participants. Blood was collected by a trained member of the research team using the Tasso-SST (Seattle, Washington, USA) device. Prior to use on participants, RTI International laboratories verified the devices were lead-free. The Tasso-SST device collected approximately 250 µg/L of blood from the deltoid region of the arm. All samples were analyzed within 30 days of collection. Lead was analyzed at RTI International laboratories via ICPMS (30).

Water sample collection and analysis

Participants collected water samples in the morning after an overnight stagnation period of at least six hours. Such "first flush" samples are intended to capture the maximum potential for lead exposure due to extended release of lead from plumbing and fixtures as water stagnates in the household water system overnight. Participants were provided with detailed oral and written instructions and two 500 mL water bottles. Participants were directed to collect the water before anyone in the household used the water. They were directed to collect cold water, and to only open the bottle for collection to reduce the risk of potential lead contamination. Once the water was collected, participants placed the water bottles in a sealed bag, which was collected by a member of the research team on the same day.

During the initial household visit, a member of the research team used a Hanna Instruments (Smithfield, RI), Model HI 8130 Combo pH/Conductivity/TDS Tester to test the pH, conductivity, and temperature of the water. Lead and other toxic heavy metals were analyzed at RTI International laboratories via ICPMS using EPA Method 200.8 (37).

Dust sample collection and analysis

A member of the research team collected up to five dust samples at the initial home visit: 1) the floor of the entry way, 2) the floor of the room the participant uses most, 3) the floor of the room where the participant sleeps, 4) the windowsill of the room where the participant sleeps, 5) the window trough of the room where the participant sleeps. Where possible, a one meter by one meter area was measured a taped off. When this area was not possible, the research team member measured and documented the area. GhostWipes® (Environmental Express, Charleston, SC) were used for dust sample collection on all surfaces. The area was completely wiped in an up-and-down motion until the full area had been sampled. When collection was complete, the researcher placed the wipe in a collection tube. Researchers wore gloves for sample collection and changed gloves between areas.

Lead and other metals were analyzed at RTI International laboratories via ICPMS with procedures the American Industrial Hygiene Association's environmental lead program at RTI (38).

Questionnaire

To understand demographic and behavioral characteristics of the participant and characteristics of the home, well, and water that may influence lead exposure risks, a research staff member administered a questionnaire. To understand the characteristics of the well, data on the well age and depth were obtained. To understand home characteristics, data regarding the home age and length of time in residence was collected. Understanding the year the home and well were built is necessary to characterize lead exposure through plumbing materials and lead-based paint. To understand potential sources of lead exposure outside of the home, data on participants' occupation and/or the school they attend was also collected. Additionally, research staff obtained information about each area of the house where a dust sample was collected, including the last time the area was cleaned and the method used to clean the area. Participants self-reported their age, date of birth, height, and weight.

Statistical analysis

A multivariable regression was performed to analyze the association between blood lead concentration and water lead concentration while controlling for other potential sources of lead exposure and for behavioral and demographic factors potentially associated with lead exposure. Chi-square tests were used to assess differences in categorical variables among participant subgroups. All statistical analyses were conducted using R.

Findings

In total, 89 participants in 75 households located in eight NC counties participated (see Figure 2). Table 1 summarizes participant demographics, water consumption behaviors, and characteristics of the households. Approximately 89% of participants reported regularly drinking water from their tap, with an average of 80% of water consumed at home coming from the tap. 70% of participants reported using a water filter. The mean age of participants was 21 years. The majority of participants were in the age category 0 years old – 8 years old, followed by the >30 age group. Approximately 61% of participants identified as white, 15% identified as American Indian, 10% identified as African American or Black, 10% identified with more than one race, 2% identified as Hispanic or Latino/a/x, and 2.3% did not report their race or ethnicity. Among participants, 38% reported having a master's degree or higher, 26% reported having a 4-year degree, 24% reported having some college, and 12% reported having a high school education or less. Among the 75 homes, 79% were built after lead paint was banned in 1978.

Table 1. Demographic, environmental, and behavioral characteristics of study participants

Characteristics of participants	
Gender	(N)(%)
Female	45 (51)
Male	44 (49)
Race	
American Indian or Alaskan Native	13 (15)
Black	9 (10)
Hispanic Latino/a	2 (2.3)
More than one race	9 (10)
White	54 (61)
Na	2 (2.3)
Age group	
0 to 8	56 (63)
9 to 14	5 (5.6)
15 to 19	1 (1.1)
20 to 29	3 (3.4)
>30	24 (27)
Na	1 (1.1)
Age (mean) (SD)	21 (25)
Characteristics of home	
County	
Alamance	2 (2.3)
Chatham	10 (11)
Durham	4 (4.5)
Hoke	1 (1.1)
Orange	7 (7.9)
Robeson	13 (15)
Union	31 (35)
Wake	21 (24)
Year home was built	
Before 1950	3 (3.4)
1950-1977	5 (5.6)
1978-1987	17 (19)
1988-1997	21 (24)
1998-2002	11 (12)
2003 or later	21 (24)
Na	11 (12)
Water filter?	
Yes	62 (70)
No	18 (20)
NA	9 (10)

Behavioral characteristics of participant	
Drink water from the tap?	
Yes	79 (89)
No	9 (10)
NA	1(1.1)
Percent of the time drink water from the tap	80 (36)
Months participant has lived in the home (mean) (SD)	90 (111)
Smoke cigarettes inside the home?	
Yes	13 (15)
No	76 (85)
Education of adult participant or parent of child participant	
High school or less	11 (12)
Some college	21 (24)
4-year college/University Degree	23 (26)
Graduate degree (e.g., M.D., J.D., Ph.D.)	34 (38)

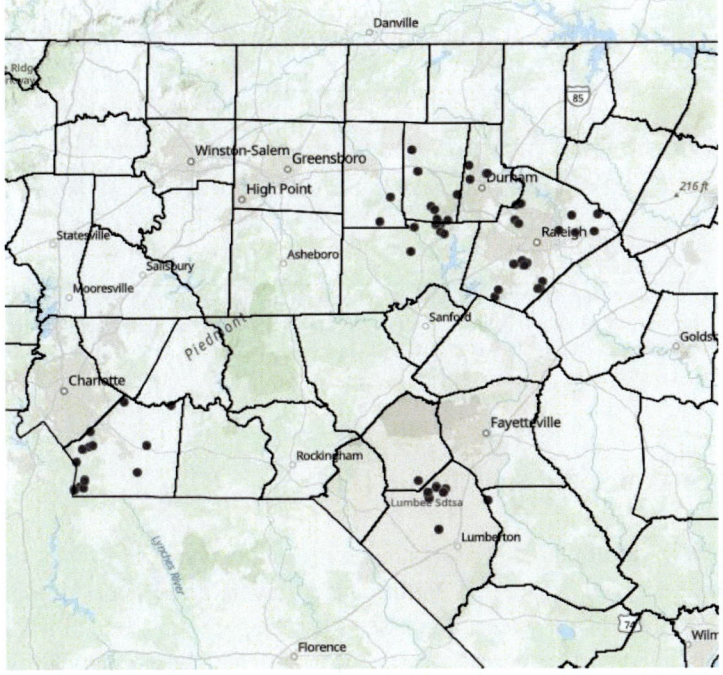

Figure 2. Locations of study participants.

Lead concentrations in blood, water and dust samples

The mean blood lead level for the study sample was 0.68 µg/dL (SD = 0.4, maximum = 2.3 µg/dL) (see Table 2, Figure 3). No participant's blood lead exceeded the CDC's blood lead reference level of concern (3.5 µg/L). The mean water lead level was 3.5 µg/L (SD = 6.5, maximum = 50). Three of the 75 households had an average water lead concentration above the EPA's action level of 15 µg/L. The mean floor lead dust concentration was 13 µg/m^2 (SD = 111, maximum 1,051). Lead dust in one home exceeded the EPA's clearance level of 108 µg/m^2 (10 µg/ft^2). The mean window lead dust concentration was 151 µg/m^2 (SD = 1,020, maximum = 8,639). Window dust in one home was above the EPA's clearance level of 1,076 µg/m^2 (100 µg/ft^2).

Table 2. Lead concentrations in collected samples

	Blood (n = 89)	Water (n = 75)	Window Dust (n = 75)	Floor Dust (n = 75)
Maximum	2.26 µg/dL	50.2 µg/dL	8639 µg/m^2	1052 µg/m^2
Mean (SD)	0.68 (0.41) µg/dL	3.49 (6.5) µg/dL	151.33 (1,020) µg/m^2	13.3 (111.3) µg/m^2
Relevant Guideline Value or Standard	3.5 µg/dL	15 µg/L	1,076 µg/m^2	108 µg/m^2

NOTE: Water and dust lead summary statistics represent averages of samples within each household. The blood lead guideline value is from CDC. The water lead guideline value represents EPA's action level for community water supplies. Dust guideline values are EPA's clearance standards for lead remediation.

Factors associated with blood lead

Blood lead was not directly associated with lead in water. However, those who filtered their well water had significantly lower blood lead compared with those who did not use water filters (see Table 3, $p < 0.05$). Use of a water filter was associated with a decrease of 32% in blood lead, when controlling for age, sex, average lead in floor dust, and whether the participant reported drinking their tap water at home. In addition, use of a filter was significantly associated with a decreased risk of the occurrence of high levels of lead in drinking water, defined as water lead about the 75th percentile for the sample (3.52 µg/L). Among participants who did not use a filter, 50% had high water lead, compared to only 16% of those who filtered their water (see Table 3, $p = 0.01$; Figure 4).

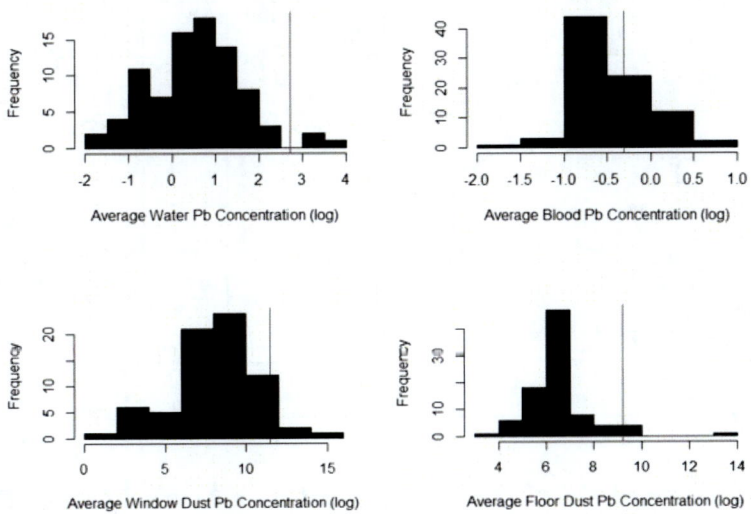

Figure 3. Lead (Pb) concentrations in water, blood, window, and floor dust samples. For water, window, and floor dust, red lines represent the EPA's action or clearance level. The red line on the blood lead histogram represents the U.S. 50th percentile of blood lead concentrations

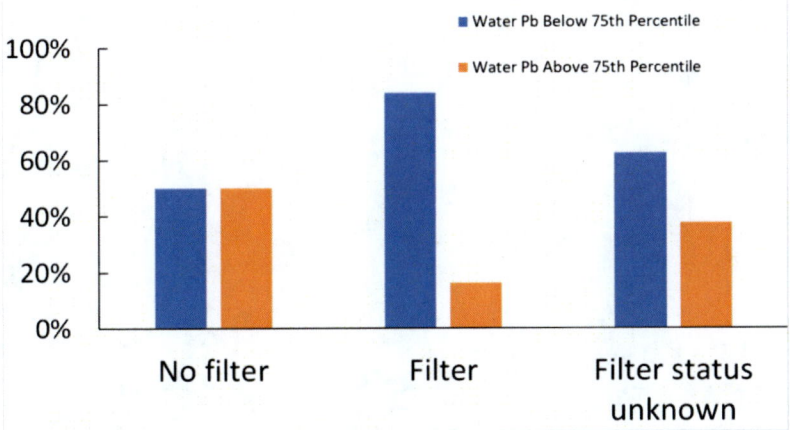

Figure 4. Participants who filtered their water were less likely to have high water lead (above the third quartile concentration for this sample, 3.5 µg/L) than those who did not have filters.

Table 3. Influence of demographic, household, and environmental factors on participant blood lead levels (log transformed)

	Coefficient	Exponentiated Coefficient	SE	t	p
(Intercept)	-1.06	0.35	0.315	-3.364	0.0012
Age	0.0075	1.0	0.002	3.601	0.00056
Sex = Male	0.11	1.1	0.100	1.142	0.26
Race = White, Asian, Latino/a, or Other (vs. African American or Native American)	-0.075	0.93	0.136	-0.551	0.58
log(Floor_Pb)	0.070	1.1	0.038	1.829	0.071
Filter Use = Unknown (vs. No)	-0.15	0.86	0.226	-0.656	0.51
Filter Use = Yes (vs. No)	-0.38	0.68	0.148	-2.591	0.011
Drink Tap Water (vs. Do Not Drink)	0.21	1.2	0.177	1.210	0.23

Regression results are based on data from 84 participants with complete data for all variables included.

We observed significant racial disparities in access to water filters. Among participants identifying as African American or Native American, 38% had a water filter, compared to 83% of those identifying as other races ($p < 0.001$) (see Figure 5).

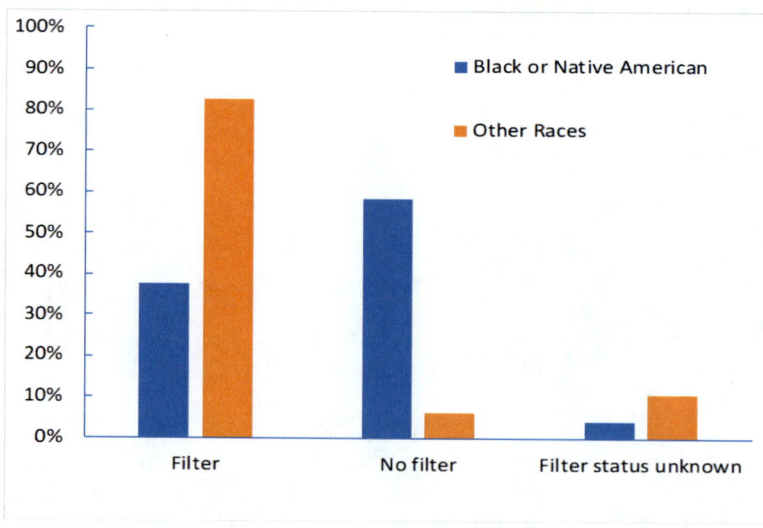

Figure 5. Black and Native Americans were less likely to own water filters than participants of other races.

Discussion

In this study, we examined blood lead levels in people who get their drinking water from a private well. Although we did not find a significant association between blood lead and water lead, our results show that use of a water filter is associated with decreased water lead levels *and* decreased blood lead levels. We also found that those who filtered their water (70% of the study participants) were significantly less likely to be exposed to high levels of lead (above the third quartile of the water lead concentration, 3.5 µg/dL) in their drinking water. Together, these results suggest that water filters remove lead from the water and therefore can effectively break the link between lead in drinking water and lead in blood. However, we found significant racial disparities in the use of water filters. Among Black and Native American participants, 38% had water filters, compared to 83% of participants from other racial groups. While this study did not explore the reason Black and Native American participants did not use a water filter, the disparity cannot be ignored. It is recommended that future studies further examine the causes of this disparity in access to safe water technology. Additionally, it is worth noting that any well used for drinking water with water lead concentrations above the EPA's action level of 15 mg/l should used filters certified to reduce lead.

Comparison to previous studies

The results of this study are consistent with previous studies suggesting that US households relying on private well water are at risk from exposure to lead in drinking water unless they install a corrosion control system (such as a whole-house acid neutralizer) or filter their water to remove lead (22, 23). Related research has found that US children relying on a private well for their drinking water have a 25% increased risk for elevated blood lead levels when compared to their counterparts who have access to regulated, municipal water systems (33). Additionally, research has found that water filters can significantly decrease lead concentrations in water sourced from private wells (39). In this study, it shows that participants who had access to a water filter were able to break the link between lead in private well water and the blood lead of those consuming the water.

Limitations

The limitations of this study include difficulty in recruiting participants from our target population. This limits the generalizability of our results as the majority of our participants were white, highly educated, and used water filters. Additionally, 37% of participants were above the age of 8. Because young children have yet to develop mature mechanisms to rid their bodies of lead quickly, our results are likely not generalizable to young children. Because water lead concentrations and blood lead concentrations may fluctuate over time, another limitation is that samples were collected at just one time point. Because only 20% of participants in our study reported not using a water filter, we have limited ability to make inferences about the associations between lead in water and lead in blood.

Conclusion

To the best of our knowledge, this is the first US study to investigate the blood lead levels in people who rely on private wells for their drinking water by collecting contemporaneous blood, water, and household dust samples. We found that using a water filter was associated with a significant decrease in exposure to lead in water and in blood lead. However, there were significant racial disparities in access to water filters, with fewerBlack and Native American participants having filters, compared to the large majority of participants of other races. It thus appears that disparities in access to safe water technology could be an important contributor to entrenched disparities in blood lead levels in the United States. Expanding access to safe water technology, either through assurance of service by an effectively managed community water system or through distribution and continuous maintenance of household water filters, could be an important step in decreasing these disparities. The use of a water filter helped prevent high levels. The majority of participants were white, highly educated, and had access to water filters. Education and race are each factors that have been shown to impact blood lead levels (34, 35). It is recommended that future studies that aim to examine the association between blood lead and water lead focus recruitment strategies to include participants with a more diverse racial and ethnic background. Additionally, it is recommended that more households that do not use a filter are included. More broadly, steps are needed to provide equitable access to water filters for households relying on private wells.

Acknowledgments

This project was financially supported by EPA Science to Achieve Results program (EPA RD-83927902-0) and the National Science Foundation (NSF CMMI-2017207).

References

[1] Lead poisoning. URL: https://www.who.int/news-room/fact-sheets/detail/lead-poisoning-and-health.
[2] Centers for Disease Control and Prevention. Populations at higher risk: Lead URL: https://www.cdc.gov/nceh/lead/prevention/populations.htm.
[3] Sorensen LC, Fox AM, Jung H, Martin EG. Lead exposure and academic achievement: evidence from childhood lead poisoning prevention efforts. J Popul Econ 2019;32(1):179–218.
[4] Goodlad JK, Marcus DK, Fulton JJ. Lead and attention-deficit/hyperactivity disorder (ADHD) symptoms: A meta-analysis. Clin Psychol Rev 2013;33(3):417–25.
[5] Needleman HL, Schell A, Bellinger D, Leviton A, Allred EN. The long-term effects of exposure to low doses of lead in childhood. An 11-year follow-up report. N Engl J Med 1990;322(2):83–8.
[6] Mansouri MT, Muñoz-Fambuena I, Cauli O. Cognitive impairment associated with chronic lead exposure in adults. Neurol Psychiatry Brain Res 2018;30:5–8.
[7] Centers for Disease Control and Prevention. Lead: Health problems caused by lead. URL: https://www.cdc.gov/niosh/topics/lead/health.html.
[8] Rosin A. The long-term consequences of exposure to lead. Isr Med Assoc J 2009;11(11):689–94.
[9] Spivey A. The weight of lead: Effects add up in adults. Environ Health Perspect 2007;115(1):A30-6.
[10] Centers for Disease Control and Prevention. National childhood blood lead surveillance data, 2021. URL: https://www.cdc.gov/nceh/lead/data/national.htm.
[11] US EPA. Protect your family from sources of lead, 2013. URL: https://www.epa.gov/lead/protect-your-family-sources-lead.
[12] US EPA. EPA history: Lead, 2013. URL: https://www.epa.gov/history/epa-history-lead.
[13] US EPA. Summary of the Safe Drinking Water Act, 2013. URL: https://www.epa.gov/laws-regulations/summary-safe-drinking-water-act.

[14] US EPA. Use of lead free pipes, fittings, fixtures, solder, and flux for drinking water, 2015. URL: https://www.epa.gov/sdwa/use-lead-free-pipes-fittings-fixtures-solder-and-flux-drinking-water.

[15] US EPA. Basic information about lead in drinking water, 2016. URL: https://www.epa.gov/ground-water-and-drinking-water/basic-information-about-lead-drinking-water.

[16] Teye SO, Yanosky JD, Cuffee Y, Weng X, Luquis R, Farace E, et al. Exploring persistent racial/ethnic disparities in lead exposure among American children aged 1-5 years: Results from NHANES 1999-2016. Int Arch Occup Environ Health 2021;94(4):723–30.

[17] Hanna-Attisha M, LaChance J, Sadler RC, Champney Schnepp A. Elevated blood lead levels in children associated with the Flint Drinking Water Crisis: A spatial analysis of risk and public health response. Am J Public Health 2016;106(2):283–90.

[18] Denchak, M. Flint Water Crisis: Everything you need to know. URL: https://www.nrdc.org/stories/flint-water-crisis-everything-you-need-know.

[19] Domestic (private) supply wells. US Geological Survey. URL: https://www.usgs.gov/mission-areas/water-resources/science/domestic-private-supply-wells?qt-science_center_objects = 0#qt-science_center_objects.

[20] US EPA. Information about public water systems, 2015. URL: https://www.epa.gov/dwreginfo/information-about-public-water-systems.

[21] Zheng Y, Flanagan SV. The case for universal screening of private well water quality in the US and testing requirements to achieve it: Evidence from arsenic. Environ Health Perspect 2017;125(8):085002.

[22] Stillo F, Gibson JM. Racial disparities in access to municipal water supplies in the American south: Impacts on children's health. In: Rubin IL, Merrick J, eds. Resilience and health. A potent dynamic. New York: Nova Science, 2018:131-56.

[23] Pieper KJ, Krometis LAH, Gallagher DL, Benham BL, Edwards M. Incidence of waterborne lead in private drinking water systems in Virginia. J Water Health 2015;13(3):897–908.

[24] Hunter B, Walker I, Lassiter R, Lassiter V, Gibson JM, Ferguson PL, et al. Evaluation of private well contaminants in an underserved North Carolina community. Sci Total Environ 2021;789:147823.

[25] Swistock BR, Clemens S, Sharpe WE, Rummel S. Water quality and management of private drinking water wells in Pennsylvania. J Environ Health 2013;75(6):60–7.

[26] Knobeloch L, Gorski P, Christenson M, Anderson H. Private drinking water quality in rural Wisconsin. J Environ Health 2013;75(7):16–20.

[27] Geiger SD, Bressler J, Kelly W, Jacobs DE, Awadalla SS, Hagston B, et al. Predictors of water lead levels in drinking water of homes with domestic wells in 3 Illinois counties. J Public Health Manag Pract 2021;27(6):567–76.

[28] Ranganathan M, Balazs C. Water marginalization at the urban fringe: environmental justice and urban political ecology across the North–South divide. Urban Geogr 2015;36(3):403–23.

[29] Joyner AM, Parnell AM. Maximizing the power of geographic information systems in racial justice. Clgh Rev 2013;47:185.
[30] Durst NJ. Municipal annexation and the selective underbounding of colonias in Texas' Lower Rio Grande Valley. Environ Plan Econ Space 2014;46(7):1699–715.
[31] Anderson MW. Cities inside out: Race, poverty, and exclusion at the urban fringe. UCLA Law Rev 2008 Jun 23. URL: https://www.uclalawreview.org/cities-inside-out-race-poverty-and-exclusion-at-the-urban-fringe/.
[32] Gibson J, Defelice N, Sebastian D, Leker H. Racial disparities in access to community water supply service in Wake County, North Carolina. Am J Public Health 2014;104:e45.
[33] Gibson JM, Fisher M, Clonch A, MacDonald JM, Cook PJ. Children drinking private well water have higher blood lead than those with city water. Proc Natl Acad Sci 2020;117(29):16898–907.
[34] Roostaei J, Colley S, Mulhern R, May AA, Gibson JM. Predicting the risk of GenX contamination in private well water using a machine-learned Bayesian network model. J Hazard Mater 2021;411:125073.
[35] MacDonald Gibson J, Iii FS, Wood E, Lockhart S, Bruine de Bruin W. Private well testing in peri-urban African-American communities lacking access to regulated municipal drinking water: A mental models approach to risk communication. Risk Anal Off Publ Soc Risk Anal 2022;42(4):799–817.
[36] Harrington JM, Young DJ, Essader AS, Sumner SJ, Levine KE. Analysis of human serum and whole blood for mineral content by ICP-MS and ICP-OES: Development of a mineralomics method. Biol Trace Elem Res 2014;160(1):132–42.
[37] Long SE, Martin TD. Determination of trace elements in waters and wastes by inductively coupled plasma - mass spectrometry: Method 200. 8. Version 4.0. Cincinnati, OH: Environmental Protection Agency, Environmental Monitoring Systems Lab, 1989. URL: https://www.osti.gov/biblio/6645038.
[38] Grunder FI. Environmental lead proficiency analytical testing (ELPAT) program. AIHA J 2003;64(1):124–7.
[39] Mulhern R, Gibson JM. Under-sink activated carbon water filters effectively remove lead from private well water for over six months, 2020. URL: https://www.rti.org/publication/under-sink-activated-carbon-water-filters-effectively-remove-lead-private-well-water.

Chapter 6

The more you know: Insights from integrated pre-visit surveys in a Pediatric Environmental Health Center

Shalini H Shah[1-4,*], DO
Alan D Woolf[1-4], MD, MPH
Kimberly Manning[2], MA, CHES
Faye Holder-Niles[3-4], MD, MPH
Bridget Tully[1-4], BS
Shelby Flanagan[2-4], MPH
Matthew C Spence[2], MPH
and Marissa Hauptman[1-4], MD, MPH

[1]Pediatric Environmental Health Center, Boston Children's Hospital, Boston, Massachusetts, United States of America
[2]Region 1 New England Pediatric Environmental Health Specialty Unit, Boston, Massachusetts, United States of America
[3]Division of General Pediatrics, Boston Children's Hospital, Boston, Massachusetts, United States of America
[4]Department of Pediatrics, Harvard Medical School, Boston, Massachusetts, United States of America

---

[*] *Correspondence:* Shalini H Shah, DO, Boston Children's Hospital, Department of Pediatrics, 300 Longwood Avenue, Boston, MA 02115, United States.
Email: shalini.shah@childrens.harvard.edu.

In: Environmental Health Disparities
Editors: I. Leslie Rubin and Joav Merrick
ISBN: 979-8-89113-487-4
© 2024 Nova Science Publishers, Inc.

Abbreviations

PEHC	Pediatric Environmental Health Center
EMR	electronic medical record
SDOH	social determinants of health
PFAS	perfluoroalkyl and polyfluoroalkyl substances

Abstract

The Pediatric Environmental Health Center (PEHC) at Boston Children's Hospital is a specialty referral clinic that provides consultation for approximately 250 patients annually. Identifying environmental hazards is key for clinical management. Exposure concerns include lead, mold, pesticides, perfluoroalkyl substances (PFAS), impaired air quality, and more. Our goal was to identify concerns and health priorities of our patient population to guide visits. A 47-question pre-visit survey was created exploring potential environmental hazards and administered prior to visits using a platform integrated into the electronic medical record (EMR). The study group was a convenience sample of patients from June 2021 to June 2022. Of 204 total visits, 101 surveys were submitted, yielding a response rate of 49.5%. 66/101 (65.3%) were surveys from initial consultations used for descriptive analysis. The majority of patients were seen for a chief complaint of lead exposure (90.1%). Most respondents had concerns about peeling paint (40.0%), and those reporting peeling paint were more likely to report additional concerns [75.0%, $p < 0.001$]. Other concerns highlighted were mold (15.2%), pests (15.2%), asbestos (10.6%), air pollution (9.1%), temperature regulation (7.6%), pesticides (6.1%), PFAS (4.5%), and formaldehyde (4.5%). A knowledge gap was identified; 45.5% (30/66) respondents responded "no" to the question asking if the Poison Center phone number was stored in their phone. This study illustrates how the implementation of a pre-visit EMR integrated survey engages families, informs clinical care, and serves as a point-of-care education tool for specific knowledge gaps. Findings will guide development of future environmental health screeners.

Introduction

Social determinants of health (SDOH) are defined as the conditions in which individuals are born, grow, live, work and play, which significantly impact health outcomes and are widely recognized in the healthcare community. SDOH include many factors such as poverty, housing and food insecurity, access to education and healthcare, immigration status, and systemic racism (1). The central tenet of the SDOH construct asks the medical and scientific community to understand and examine the conditions in which children are living, in the hopes that detecting and addressing these components can serve as an opportunity to reduce health disparities and improve long-term health outcomes. Despite this goal of understanding the livelihoods of our patients and life conditions affecting their communities, the environmental aspects of SDOH are often overlooked in clinical practice.

Environmental pollution is widespread and continues to contaminate our air, water, and soil, and the public health community's understanding of the health risks posed by these exposures is sound, robust, and evolving. Lifetime exposure to environmental pollutants has been linked to low birth weight, asthma, cancer, and neurodevelopmental disorders (2). Exposure to air pollution has a variety of short and long-term health effects, which may be experienced as symptoms of cough, wheezing, and shortness of breath with high rates of hospitalization. Cumulative impacts of respiratory diseases can be lifelong, such as the development of chronic asthma, chronic obstructive pulmonary disease, pulmonary insufficiency, and cardiovascular disorders in adulthood (2). Water contamination exposes vulnerable children to toxic heavy metals such as lead, arsenic, mercury, and cadmium, with an increased risk of health consequences including developmental/neurocognitive/behavioral disorders, respiratory illness, cardiovascular disease, and cancer (3). Of these heavy metals, lead is the most common and most studied neurotoxin with a large body of evidence that links exposure to negative impacts on brain function and child development, causing learning and behavior impairment (4). The most common exposure source is via ingestion of lead dust from deteriorating lead-based paint, which is more prevalent in older housing and housing in poor condition (5). Resultant lead exposure and the related neurodevelopmental health concerns are key examples of the health consequences of environmental injustice and systemic inequity (6). While these are well-studied examples interlinking the presence of environmental hazards and health outcomes, there are innumerable emerging exposures in our environments that likely contribute to adverse health outcomes, though the specific impacts may not yet be understood.

Children are an especially vulnerable subset of the population to environmental threats due in part to their unique physiological, social, and environmental factors; they have higher respiratory rates, have impaired thermoregulatory conditioning, and carry greater exposure risk through demographics affecting their housing, school, and outdoor play and are reliant on caregivers (7). Children of low income and minority communities experience a disproportionately high burden given their increased exposure with limited resources available for adaptation. This can be amplified by barriers to access to solutions because of poverty, environmental racism, and systemic inequity (6, 8). The compounding effects of social and economic disadvantage, amplified by systemic racism and environmental injustice have been described as a cycle of child health disparities (see Figure 1) and contribute to poor health outcomes for disadvantaged children (9).

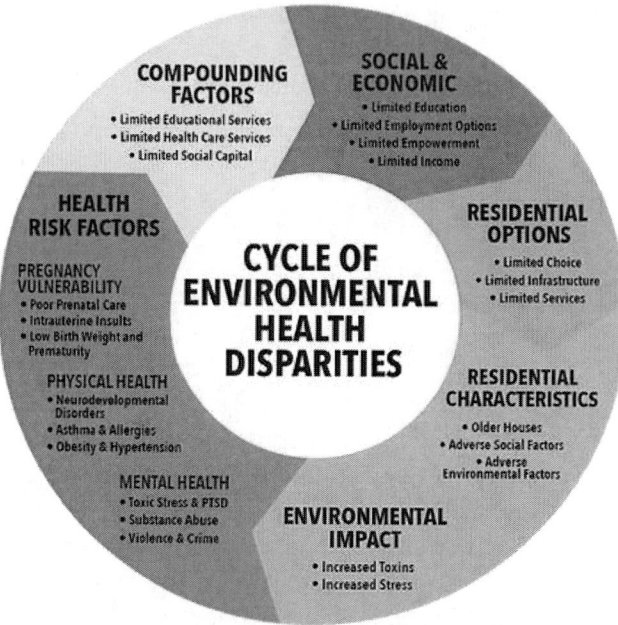

Figure 1. The cycle of environmental health disparities (9).

Despite the robust evidence showing how environmental hazards impact child health and long-term outcomes, most pediatric healthcare providers do not integrate environmental health assessments into their clinical practice. There are multiple barriers to integrating environmental health into practice, including the time constraints of visits, lack of provider knowledge or confidence in discussing and addressing environmental health concerns with families, and limited resources available for positive findings such as community-based partnerships, educational handouts, and referral programs for addressing housing or environmental concerns directly. The lack of recognizing and incorporating environmental considerations into clinical practice can be paralleled to the early phases of integrating the role of SDOH in medical care. Integration of SDOH into practice is often achieved using screening tools prior to or as a part of the clinical encounter. Though several SDOH screeners exist, a systematic review of 11 SDOH screeners in pediatrics revealed the environmental questions are limited to housing stability and neighborhood crime (10). To our knowledge, a well-integrated or validated environmental health screening tool does not currently exist for routine use in pediatric practice.

The Pediatric Environmental Health Center (PEHC) at Boston Children's Hospital is an urban specialty clinic that sees, on average, two hundred fifty patients annually, the majority of whom present with elevated blood lead levels or lead poisoning. Other clinical concerns prompting evaluation include mold or pesticide exposure, potential hazards from air and water quality concerns, and heavy metal exposures such as lead, arsenic, or mercury. Further, there is an emerging level of medical concern regarding exposure to perfluoroalkyl and polyfluoroalkyl substances (PFAS) such as its role as an endocrine disruptor, altering immune and thyroid function, contributing to liver and renal disease, negative reproductive and developmental outcomes, as well as being linked to renal and testicular cancers (12). Providers are typically allotted thirty to sixty minutes to conduct their consultation visits, although the reality of face-to-face time with patients and families is often much less, due to inconsistent start times with delayed patient arrival, time required for check-in, registration, and preceding clinical assistant assessments such as vital signs +/- connecting with an interpreter if needed. These barriers limit the depth to which environmental health histories can explore additional hazards that may be present but not directly linked or recognized as relevant to the chief complaint. Lack of standardization of electronic medical records (EMR) and approach to taking an environmental health history can lead to gaps in care. Relying on retrospective chart review where pertinent historical information may be present in different areas (including but not limited to the demographics section, provider clinical notes, non-EMR integrated intake documentation led by schedulers) can lead to providers missing key environmental needs or hazards identified by families on an individual case level. This also makes large-scale analysis for population management more challenging than if this information was collated in a database.

The aim of this project was to develop a pre-visit survey to improve clinical care provided at the PEHC, increase environmental health literacy, and identify other environmental hazards within a population seen primarily for lead poisoning to provide more comprehensive care and inform center initiatives. In consideration of the cycle of health disparities outlined by the Break the Cycle of Children's Environmental Health Disparities Program, lead exposure and lead poisoning can be viewed within the cycle framework in that limited social and economic capital leads to inadequate residential options that are more likely to contain lead hazards; this environmental exposure directly impacts the health and growth of the developing child (see Figure 1). This initiative aims to break this intergenerational cycle by detecting residential, community, and environmental hazards that contribute to negative health outcomes and providing clinical intervention(s) to ultimately decrease the burden of adverse childhood health outcomes (see Figure 2). It serves as a foundation upon which to develop future environmental health screening tools for use more broadly in pediatrics.

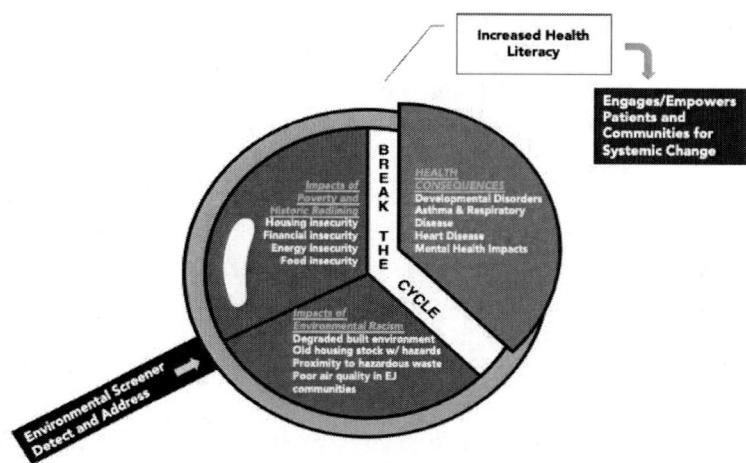

Figure 2. Environmental health screening as a tool to break the cycle of health disparities.

Our study

This project was conducted in multiple phases. The initial steps included a review of the literature to develop a broad understanding of current screening tools utilized in pediatric care such as screening for domestic or intimate partner violence, depression, and other SDOH (10). This information provided a foundation and knowledge base to inform the development of the environmental survey used in this study. The primary environmental medicine team, consisting of pediatric environmental health clinical faculty and health educators, then developed a questionnaire by using the electronic medical record integrated pre-visit survey platform, Tonic for Health. This platform allows for questionnaires to be sent electronically to patients and families via email prior to their scheduled clinical consultation. This questionnaire was pretested and modified after focus group review. The finalized version included a total of 47 questions spanning a wide range of environmental health topics. It was administered to a convenience sample of patients prior to their scheduled visits in the PEHC from June 18, 2021 through June 18, 2022 (one calendar year). Surveys were administered to all scheduled patients irrespective of initial consultation versus follow-up visits. Families received the intake survey by email five days prior to their appointment with automated reminders three days and again 24 hours prior to the visit. Individual survey responses were automatically uploaded into the electronic medical record to allow provider review prior to or during clinical encounters to address needs during the visit as appropriate. Aggregate data was extracted at the end of the study period through the Tonic for Health database and reviewed using descriptive statistical analysis. Duplicate surveys from follow-up visits were excluded from analysis. This project qualifies as a quality improvement initiative by the Boston Children's Hospital Institutional Review Board.

Findings

In the one-year study period, there were a total of 204 clinical encounters in the PEHC. Clinic demographics show that nearly 25% of families seen in the center reside in high-risk areas for lead exposure or poisoning as defined by the 2020 Annual Childhood Lead Poisoning Surveillance Report for Massachusetts (11). Approximately 20% of patients seen in the center identify as non-white, 13% report English is not their primary language and most patients (53%) are on public insurance. Of the 204 visits in the study period, 101 surveys were completed, yielding a response rate of 49.5%. Of the 101 surveys completed, 66 were unique patients or initial visits (65.3%) and the remainder of submitted surveys were follow-up visits (34.7%, 35/101). Chart review of these 66 encounters revealed that 90.9% (60/66) of these patients had a chief complaint of lead exposure. The following results and analysis are based upon review of the survey data collected from these unique patient encounters (n = 66).

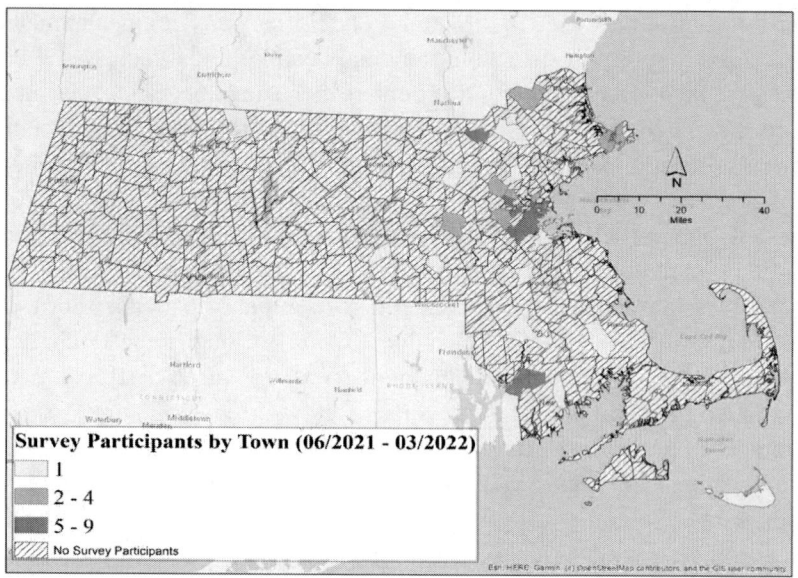

Figure 3. Geographic distribution of survey respondents.

There was a geographic distribution of a total of 37 towns in Massachusetts and two in Rhode Island (see Figure 3). As seen in Table 1, housing ownership distribution indicated the majority of patients owned their home at 51.5% (34/66) as primary owners (owner-occupied), and 6.1% (4/66) owned by extended family. The remainder 37.9% (25/66) rent their residence; 4.4% refused to answer this question (4/66). A total of 44/66 respondents (66.7%) reported lead inspection had been performed in their home, 25.0% (11/44) of this subgroup reported multiple forms of inspection (Department of Public Health, private inspector and/or lead test kits). Of those who reported inspections, 93.2% (41/44) reported that hazards were identified (options: lead in paint, dust/soil, air, water, disposal of lead wastes, other with free text option). Respondents identified an array of concerns as illustrated in Figure 4. These concerns identified, in descending order, were peeling paint (40.0%, 24/66), mold (15.2%, 10/66), pests (15.2%, 10/66), asbestos (10.6%, 7/66), air pollution (9.1%, 6/66), temperature regulation (7.6%, 5/66), pesticides (6.1%, 4/66), PFAS (4.5%, 3/66), and formaldehyde (4.5%, 3/66). 75.0% (18/24) of those with peeling paint (a lead-related concern) identified additional environmental concerns (p < 0.001). For the educational question inquiring if the Poison Center telephone number was stored in the respondent's phone, 45.5% (30/66) answered no.

Table 1. Patient demographics by reported peeling paint concerns

	Totals	No Peeling Paint Concerns	Peeling Paint Concerns	P value
	N = 66 surveys	N = 42 surveys	N = 24 surveys	
Visit Chief Complaint				<0.012
Non-Lead Exposure Concerns	6 (9.1%)	1 (2.4%)	5 (20.8%)	
Lead Exposure Concerns	60 (90.9%)	41 (97.6%)	19 (79.2%)	
Housing Type				0.54
Apartment	20 (30.3%)	12 (28.6%)	8 (33.3%)	
Multi-Family	12 (18.2%)	9 (21.4%)	3 (12.5%)	
Single Family	32 (48.5%)	19 (45.2%)	13 (54.2%)	
Unknown, Refuse to Answer, Skipped	2 (3.0%)	2 (4.8%)	0 (0.0%)	
Housing Ownership				0.26
Owner-Occupied	34 (51.5%)	23 (54.8%)	11 (45.8%)	
Owned by Extended Family	4 (6.1%)	4 (9.5%)	0 (0.0%)	
Rental	25 (37.9%)	13 (31.0%)	12 (50.0%)	
Unknown, Refuse to Answer, Skipped	3 (4.6%)	2 (4.8%)	1 (4.2%)	
Year Built				0.42
Pre 1900	14 (21.2%)	8 (19.1%)	6 (25.0%)	
1900-1950	20 (30.3%)	11 (26.2%)	9 (37.5%)	
1950-1978	9 (13.6%)	5 (11.9%)	4 (16.7%)	
1978-2000	5 (7.6%)	5 (11.9%)	0 (0.0%)	
Post 2000s	1 (1.5%)	1 (2.4%)	0 (0.0%)	
Unknown, Refuse to Answer, Skipped	17 (25.8%)	12 (28.6%)	5 (11.9%)	
Lead Inspection Performed				0.62
No	7 (10.6%)	5 (11.9%)	2 (8.3%)	
Yes	44 (66.7%)	29 (69.1%)	15 (62.5%)	
Unknown	15 (22.7%)	8 (19.1%)	7 (29.2%)	
Additional Environmental Concerns Reported				<0.001
No	42 (63.6%)	36 (85.7%)	6 (14.3%)	
Yes	24 (36.4%)	6 (25.0%)	18 (75.0%)	

Discussion

This pre-visit environmental survey was created by our center to better understand the scope of environmental hazards to which our patients and families are exposed. Results from our survey illustrated a broad range of priorities and key environmental concerns within our patient population (see Figure 4). Although the Pediatric Environmental Health Center primarily sees patients for lead exposure and poisoning, findings from our pre-visit survey demonstrate that families with peeling paint/lead-related concerns (75.0%) are more likely to have additional environmental concerns ($p < 0.001$) compared to those without concerns about peeling paint (see Table 1). This is significant because although these patients may be referred for their lead exposure, there is the potential that other environmental hazards are present in their home that could be impacting their health. An unexpected finding was that those who did not report peeling paint concerns were in fact more likely to have a chief complaint related to lead exposure ($p < 0.012$, Table 1). We hypothesize this may be because families who do not have visible peeling paint may be less aware of the presence of lead in their home environment, and thus unable to address it. This may lead to elevated lead levels prompting referral to our clinic. This information offers an opportunity for providers to better identify families at risk for other environmental hazards and provide more comprehensive care through anticipatory guidance. The survey also demonstrated a large percentage of PEHC families rent their primary residence vs owner-occupied (37.9% vs 51.5% respectively). An understanding of the ownership status is critical in the field of environmental health as management strategies are often impacted by who is primarily responsible for the remediation of the residence and the financial burden that may accompany these needs. Being able to track this data in our patient population aids our ability to inform initiatives within our center to help support patients and families in navigating these complexities as well as influence environmental health and housing advocacy on a broader level for environmental justice.

One of our survey questions specifically asked if the Poison Center number was stored in the respondent's device. If they stated no, it automatically provided this information within the survey platform using "branching logic" (see Figure 5). The number was provided along with instructions to save it in their device so that it would be readily available in the future in case of emergency". A large portion of respondents reported they did not have this information (45.5%) and were thus directed to this point-of-care education. To our knowledge, this is a unique feature of our screening tool, as other surveys may elucidate needs or concerns but addressing these findings is typically deferred to the provider at the clinical encounter instead of within the survey itself.

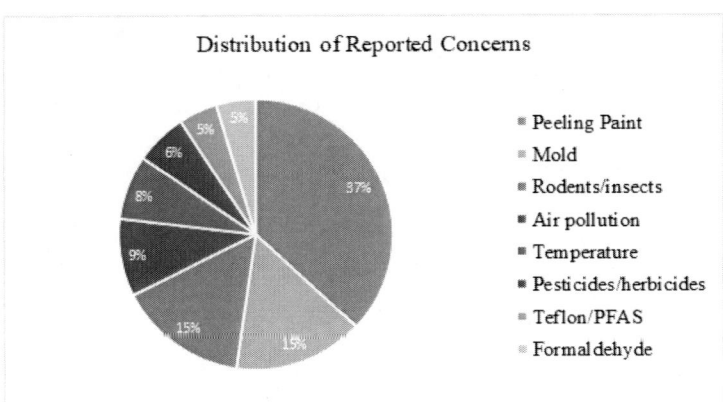

Figure 4. Distribution of reported concerns.

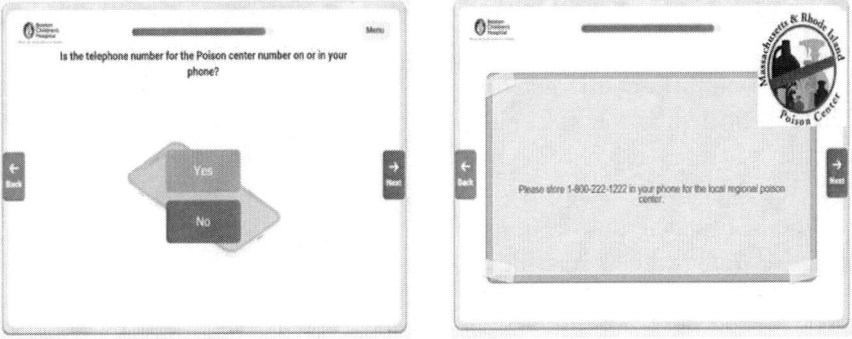

Figure 5. Tonic for health platform question sample with paired education.

Notably, PFAS was one of the least reported concerns by the study population at 4.5% despite growing evidence and national concern about health impacts of chronic PFAS exposure (12). Environmental exposures to potentially toxic chemicals like PFAS that are reported less frequently may be due to a lack of awareness on the population to the risks they may pose to human health. Analysis of lesser reported concerns and using this model of "branching logic" education in future surveys may be an opportunity to increase environmental health literacy by increasing awareness of children's exposure to potential environmental hazards. Given that improved environmental health literacy has a role in illness prevention "by raising awareness of risks from environmental factors and by providing approaches that individuals and communities can take to avoid, mitigate, or reduce such exposures," the use of an environmental health screener to increase awareness and literacy is significant (13). Further, identifying gaps in our patient population's understanding of different environmental hazards, such as PFAS and other contaminants, is useful to inform future educational outreach initiatives of our center, in hopes of increasing awareness and adaptation to different environmental health threats.

Conclusion

Results from this study show that pre-visit integrated electronic survey implementation helps engage families prior to visits and better direct anticipatory guidance to self-identified concerns. This tool demonstrated its ability to serve as a unique point-of-care platform for immediate education tailored to specific knowledge gaps. Findings from this survey can serve as a foundation for the development of further environmental health screening practices and inform a targeted screening approach that can incorporate the needs identified by families, paired with educational materials and provider resources to address identified limitations.

Generalizability of this work is limited by the convenience population in a single subspecialty environmental health clinic in a large academic center. Response rate and percentage of patients identifying environmental concerns may be influenced by this being a specialty clinic and thus families being more prepared and willing to respond to environmental screening and more sensitive questions about their home environment. This survey was only administered in English and thus may not capture the needs of our non-English speaking families and the diverse patient population seen at the Pediatric Environmental Health Center. Follow-up visit surveys were excluded from our analysis, which could lead to underestimation of hazards if patients/families reported new concerns at follow-up visits. Denial of certain environmental health hazards may be confounded by limitations of environmental health literacy and population understanding/awareness of these topics. Limitations in implementation for broader clinical practice include the length of survey serving as an obstacle both for family completion but also provider review, provider/patient understanding of environmental exposures and the role they play in child health and disease management, and limited resources available if needs are identified.

Despite these limitations, this study illustrates how the implementation of a pre-visit EMR-integrated survey engages families before visits, informs clinical care, and can serve as a point-of-care education for specific knowledge gaps. Our study confirmed a family's willingness to complete a pre-visit survey regarding details of the child's home environment prior to their scheduled specialty clinic visit. Our findings documented that, while the child was usually referred for a single environmental health hazard, a written pre-visit survey often revealed other health concerns that could (and should) also be addressed during the office visit. And though this tool was used in a specialty center, a pre-visit questionnaire similar to this may also be helpful to community pediatricians and community health centers, who serve larger numbers of vulnerable patients at risk of environmental exposures but may not have access to subspecialty care as readily available. A tool like this can be a source of education for both providers and patients in that asking about potential environmental exposures they may not otherwise consider can raise awareness that these factors may be influencing the child's health. It could also assist in directing patients to community resources for hazard mitigation. Findings from this effort will guide development of future environmental health screeners.

Acknowledgments

The preparation for this project and manuscript review was supported by the Break the Cycle of Health Disparities Program of the Southeast PEHSU at Emory University and Break the Cycle of Health Disparities, Inc.

Dr Shah's work is supported (in part) by contract # 21W201300122 from the Massachusetts Department of Public Health associated with the Appletree Grant (Component 2) sponsored by the Centers for Disease Control and Prevention, Atlanta GA.

Drs Shah, Woolf, Hauptman, Ms Manning, Tully, Flanagan and Mr Spence are also supported (in part) by the cooperative agreement award number FAIN: NU61TS000296 with the Centers for Disease Control and Prevention/Agency for Toxic Substances and Disease Registry (CDC/ATSDR). The US Environmental Protection Agency (EPA) supports the PEHSUs by providing partial funding to CDC/ATSDR through an Inter-Agency Agreement. The findings and conclusions presented have not been formally disseminated by CDC/ATSDR or EPA and should not be construed to represent any agency determination or policy. Use of trade names that may be mentioned is for identification only and does not imply endorsement by the CDC/ATSDR or EPA. Dr. Hauptman is also supported by grants from the National Institutes of Health/National Institute of Environmental Health Sciences K23 ES031663 during the conduct of the study.

Disclosure statements

The authors have no financial relationships relevant to this article to disclose. The authors have no conflicts of interest to disclose.

References

[1] Ragavan MI, Marcil LE, Garg A. Climate change as a social determinant of health. Pediatrics 2020;145(5):e20193169.
[2] Landrigan PJ, Fuller R, Fisher S, Suk WA, Sly P, Chiles TC, et al. Pollution and children's health. Sci Total Environ 2019;650(Pt 2):2389–94.
[3] Eze IC, Schaffner E, Fischer E, Schikowski T, Adam M, Imboden M, et al. Long-term air pollution exposure and diabetes in a population-based Swiss cohort. Environ Int 2014; 70:95–105. doi: 10.1016/j.envint.2014.05.014.
[4] Sanders T, Liu Y, Buchner V, Tchounwou PB. Neurotoxic effects and biomarkers of lead exposure: A review. Rev Environ Health 2009;24(1):15–46.
[5] Osman MA, Yang F, Massey IY. Exposure routes and health effects of heavy metals on children. Biometals 2019;32(4):563–73.
[6] Whitehead LS, Buchanan SD. Childhood lead poisoning: A perpetual environmental justice issue? J Public Health Man 2019;25(1):S115–20.
[7] Chance GW, Harmsen E. Children are different: Environmental contaminants and children's health. C J Public Health 1998;89(Suppl 1):S10–5.
[8] Dignam T, Kaufmann RB, LeStourgeon L, Brown MJ. Control of lead sources in the United States, 1970-2017: Public health progress and current challenges to eliminating lead exposure. J Public Health Man 2019;25(1):S13–22.
[9] Break the Cycle of Health Disparities: Atlanta, GA: Break the cycle program. URL: https://www.breakthecycleprogram.org/.
[10] Sokol R, Austin A, Chandler C, Byrum E, Bousquette J, Lancaster C, et al. Screening Children for social determinants of health: A systematic review. Pediatrics 2019;144(4):e20191622.
[11] Annual screening and blood lead level reports and high-risk community lists, 2021. URL: https://www.mass.gov/lists/annual-screening-and-blood-lead-level-reports-and-high-risk-community-lists.

[12] Fenton SE, Ducatman A, Boobis A, DeWitt JC, Lau C, Ng C, et al. Per- and polyfluoroalkyl substance toxicity and human health review: Current state of knowledge and strategies for informing future research. Environ Toxicol Chem 2021;40(3):606–30.

[13] Finn S, O'Fallon L. The emergence of environmental health literacy—From its roots to its future potential. Environ Health Persp 2017;125(4):495–501.

Chapter 7

Increasing maternal education modifies the relationship between maternal disorders during pregnancy and later life positive child health among individuals born extremely preterm

Margaret Pinder[*]
University of North Carolina at Chapel Hill, Gillings School of Global Public Health, Department of Environmental Health Sciences, Chapel Hill, North Carolina, United States of America

Abstract

The extremely low gestational age newborn (ELGAN) study collected data from over 1,506 infants from fourteen hospitals born at 28 weeks' gestation or earlier. At the time of birth, data was collected about maternal health conditions, including pre-pregnancy diabetes, obesity, hypertension and asthma. Follow-up studies were conducted when these individuals were two, ten, and fifteen years old and among the data collected were social and environmental variables, including maternal education. A positive child health index (PCHI) has been developed in order to evaluate adverse health outcomes in later life for ELGANs and to identify antecedents of positive health in childhood. This index was calculated at both the 10-year and 15-year follow-up interviews, and it is known that maternal health conditions at birth can influence PCHI among

---

[*] **Correspondence:** Rebecca C Fry, PhD, The Institute for Environmental Health Solutions, Department of Environmental Sciences and Engineering, Gillings School of Global Public Health, The University of North Carolina at Chapel Hill, Chapel Hill, NC, United States. Email: rfry@unc.edu.

In: Environmental Health Disparities
Editors: I. Leslie Rubin and Joav Merrick
ISBN: 979-8-89113-487-4
© 2024 Nova Science Publishers, Inc.

ELGANs at age 10. The aim of this project was to determine if changes in a maternal education between birth and age 15 years moderate the relationship between maternal health conditions and positive child health at age 15 years.

Introduction

Extremely low gestational age newborns (ELGANs), who are those born prior to 28 weeks' gestation, experience an increased risk of adverse developmental and health outcomes at birth and in subsequent years, as they age. At birth, these adverse outcomes can include cerebral white matter damage, lung disorders, intestinal disorders, retinal disorders, as well as systemic inflammatory conditions. In later life, adverse health outcomes can include neurodevelopmental disorders such as cerebral palsy, epilepsy, autism, and other neurological impairments. For example, at 10 years of age, in the ELGAN study cohort off children, 25% had moderate-to-severe cognitive impairment, 11.4% had cerebral palsy, 7.6% had epilepsy, 7.1% had autism spectrum disorder, and 4.9% had severe motor impairment (1). A positive child health index (PCHI) has been developed in order to evaluate adverse health outcomes in later life for ELGANs, according to a continuous model that is fairly homogeneous and takes into account multiple disorders (2). Among ELGANs, the PCHI has been associated with adverse maternal health conditions such as obesity being associated with a lower PCHI (worse health) at age 10 (1). It is currently unknown if social determinants of health could modify this existing relationship, and this study seeks to answer this question by focusing on maternal education at birth and age 15 years.

Participants for the ELGAN study were first recruited from 14 hospitals in five different states (Connecticut, Illinois, Massachusetts, Michigan and North Carolina) in 2002 and follow up studies were conducted at ages 2, 10, and 15 years. A strength of this cohort is its longitudinal design and the availability of data on pre-, peri-, and early postnatal exposure that support research on the developmental origins of disease. Although the sample size is dependent on follow up participation, the original study has been very valuable for its role in illustrating the relationship between pre- and perinatal inflammation and later-life developmental outcomes among ELGANs (1, 2). Although it is long known that children born extremely premature are at increased risk for adverse health outcomes at birth and in later life, there has been a recent focus on factors at birth associated with positive child health in later life.

Recently the ELGAN study has established the PCHI for assessing positive child health based on 11 adverse outcomes: asthma, visual impairment, hearing impairment, gross motor function impairment, epilepsy, attention deficit/hyperactivity disorder, anxiety, depression, cognitive impairment, autism, and obesity. Of note is that 32% of the cohort had none of these 11 adverse outcomes at age 10 years (1). This index was used to evaluate the relationship between positive child health and quality of life among ELGANs. Using the PCHI, linkages between positive child health at age 10 years and antecedents at birth, including maternal health conditions, were evaluated. Pre-pregnancy socioeconomic status, maternal pre-pregnancy asthma, maternal asthma during pregnancy, maternal treatment with asthma medication during pregnancy, maternal consumption of aspirin during pregnancy, and maternal obesity were associated with lower PCHI at age 10 years, indicating poorer health (1).

Gestational age has a significant impact on academic achievement-test scores, but this effect can be moderated by maternal SES and education level (3). In a study comparing 58 ELGANS to 171 preterm infants (≥28- < 34 weeks), 288 late preterm infants (≥34- < 37 weeks), and 967 term infants (≥37- < 42 weeks), prematurity was associated with a significant decrease in mathematics scores (3). Among all gestational age categories, high SES (defined as private insurance) and high maternal education (defined as any postsecondary education) were associated with higher scores on literacy and mathematics assessments. Furthermore, the negative impact of low SES and low maternal education on test scores among ELGANs diminished over time for literacy, but remained constant from grade 3 to grade 8 for mathematics scores (3).

Initially, we hypothesized that adverse maternal health conditions would be associated with a lower PCHI at 15 years of age, as was found at age 10 years. In the current study, we also evaluated the hypothesis that socioeconomic status moderates the relationship between maternal health conditions and child PCHI at 15 years. We hypothesized that positive changes in socioeconomic status will lessen the negative impacts that maternal health conditions have on a child's health.

Our study

The extremely low gestational age newborn (ELGAN) Study is an observational study of the risk of structural and functional neurologic disorders in extremely preterm infants. During the years 2002-2004, women delivering before 28 weeks' gestation in 11 cities in five states were invited to enroll in the study. A total of 1,506 infants, born to 1,249 mothers, were enrolled and 1,198 survived to age 10 years (79.5%). Among survivors, 1,102 (91.9%) participated in a 2-year assessment, and 889 (74.2%) were evaluated at ten years (4). At age 15 years, we attempted to enroll all surviving members of the ELGAN cohort (n = 1,198 alive at ten years). A total of 700 adolescents (58% of surviving cohort members) were evaluated at age 15 years. All procedures for this study were approved by the institutional review boards of all participating institutions.

Maternal and newborn characteristics

Maternal age, education, marital status, eligibility for government-provided medical care insurance (e.g., Medicaid), and racial and ethnic identity were self-reported. Maternal IQ was assessed with the Kaufman Brief Intelligence Test – 2 (KBIT-2) nonverbal subscale at the 10-year visit. This was done in order to approximate the heritable component of child IQ; however, it is important to note that maternal IQ does not necessarily reflect genetic components of cognitive function because of the influences of early childhood education and other social and economic factors.

The gestational age estimates were based on a hierarchy of the quality of available information. Most desirable were estimates based on the dates of embryo retrieval or intrauterine insemination or fetal ultrasound before the 14th week (62%). When these were not available, reliance was placed sequentially on a fetal ultrasound at 14 or more weeks (29%), LMP without fetal ultrasound (7%), and gestational age recorded in the log of the neonatal intensive care unit (1%). The birth weight Z-score is the number of standard deviations the infant's birth weight is above or below the median weight of infants at the same gestational age in a standard data set. Bronchopulmonary dysplasia was defined as receiving supplemental O_2 at 36 weeks post-conceptual age and was also termed "chronic lung disease". White matter damage, or white matter injury, was defined as the presence of both periventricular echolucency and moderate or severe ventriculomegaly.

Procedures at 15 years

Child measures were selected to provide the most comprehensive assessment of neurocognitive and academic function obtainable in a single testing session in order to maximize participation and data collection. While the child was tested and additional educational measures were assessed, the parent or caregiver completed questionnaires regarding the child's medical and neurological status and behavioral outcomes.

Positive child health measures

Participating families completed study visits during which developmental and medical outcomes were assessed. As previously described (2), at age 10 years, clinicians assessed 11 outcomes: cognitive function (School-Age Differential Ability Scales-II Verbal and Nonverbal Reasoning scales) (5); blindness (uncorrectable functional blindness in both eyes) (6); hearing (use of hearing aid, cochlear implant, or special services for hearing impaired person) (6); gross motor function (Gross Motor Function Classification System) (5); epilepsy (structured interview reviewed by two epileptologists) (7); autism (Social Communication Questionnaire Autism Diagnostic Interview–Revised, Autism Diagnostic Observation Schedule, v.2) (8-10); attention-deficit/hyperactivity disorder, anxiety and depression (Child Symptom Inventory, Parent and Teacher Checklist, 4th ed.) (11-13); asthma (medical provider's diagnosis); and obesity (BMI > 95th percentile based on CDC growth charts). At age 15 years, all the assessments were repeated, except for the ones that we assumed to persist between 10 and 15 years (blindness, hearing, gross motor function and autism). The PCHI score of 100% was assigned to teenagers having none of the 11 adverse outcomes measured.

Obesity and overweight (anthropometric data)

Weight and height were obtained by study personnel. Body mass index (BMI) was then calculated using the following formula: BMI = Weight (in kilograms)/Height (in meters)/Height (in meters). BMI Z-scores and percentiles for age and sex were then derived centrally by the study statistician, using the Statistical Analysis Software program based on current CDC growth charts. A BMI centile between 85 and just less than 95 was considered overweight and a 15-year BMI centile of 95 or above was considered obese.

Data analysis

To determine change in maternal education between birth and age 15, years of education were scaled as 1, 2, 3, 4, and 5, which correspond to years of education: < 12, 12, 13-15,16, and >16, respectively. Maternal education change was defined as any difference between maternal education status at the birth of the infant and the child at age 15 years of age, assuming that maternal education status could not decrease. To determine PCHI at 15 years of age in the ELGAN cohort and evaluate changes in PCHI score from age 10 to 15 years the following analysis plan was adopted: PCHI at age 15 years was calculated employing the same approach used to derive PCHI at age 10 years (2). In summary, a PCHI score of 100% was assigned to teenagers having none of the 11 adverse outcomes measured. PCHI score decreased by 9.1% (100/11 = 9.1) for each reported adverse outcome.

This study first sought to evaluate the relationship between maternal health conditions and children's health at age 15 years by modeling PCHI as a continuous outcome and regressing this outcome on each maternal condition. The resulting beta values represent the difference in PCHI between study participants whose mother had the particular health condition and those whose mother did not. Subsequently, changes in modifiable SES variables were evaluated, beginning with maternal education. Finally, the regression was repeated in subsets of the cohort, organized according to change in maternal education (classified as either no change or positive change). This regression accounted for the following confounding variables: sex, gestational age in days, birthweight z-score, public insurance status, and maternal education status, which were chosen because they were confounders from the 10-year PCHI analysis that were associated with the exposures and outcomes of interest in this study (1).

Findings

The sample size for this study, representing the subjects from the initial study who returned for the 15-year-old follow-up was 694 (57.8% of survivors at

10-year-follow-up). Table 1 compares the demographic characteristics of the surviving members of the ELGAN cohort with the demographic characteristics of those who returned for the 15-year evaluation. The percentage of participating children whose mothers who had completed high school increased between birth and age 15 years and the percentage of mothers covered by public insurance decreased.

46% of children who returned for follow-up were born between 25- and 26-weeks gestational age, and 33% were born at 27 weeks gestational age. Most follow-up participants were male. Among the entire follow-up cohort at age 15 years, maternal education at the child's birth was at least some college for 63% of participants, and 35% of mothers had single marital status at the time of birth. 387 mothers, or approximately 60% (57.9%) of the subset that returned for the 15-year-follow-up had no change in their education, and the remaining mothers (approximately 40%) had a positive change in their education over that 15-year period, which is impressive.

The study next examined whether this change in an SES variable affected the relationship between PCHI at age 15 years and maternal health at birth (see Table 3). As hypothesized, maternal obesity at birth was associated with worse child PCHI at age 15 years. Among children whose mothers experienced no change in years of education between the child's birth and age 15, the adjusted difference in PCHI associated with maternal obesity was -4.6 (95% CI = -6.6, -2.7; p = 1.0E-4). Among mothers who completed additional years of education between their child's birth and age 15, the adjusted difference in PCHI associated with maternal obesity was -2.7 (95% CI = -6.2, 0.75; p = 0.15).

As hypothesized, maternal diabetes was associated with worse child PCHI at age 15 years. Among children whose mothers experienced no change in years of education between the child's birth and age 15 years, the adjusted difference in PCHI associated with maternal pre-pregnancy diabetes was -5.6 (95% CI = -10.2, -1.1; p = 0.03). Among mothers who completed additional years of education between their child's birth and age 15 years, the adjusted difference in PCHI associated with maternal diabetes was 3.7 (95% CI = -12.8, 5.4; p = 0.43).

As hypothesized, maternal asthma at birth was associated with worse child PCHI at age 15 years. Among children whose mothers experienced no change in years of education between the child's birth and age 15 years, the adjusted difference in PCHI associated with maternal asthma was -4.3 (95% CI = -6.9, -1.7; p = 0.005). Among mothers who completed additional years of education between their child's birth and age 15 years, the adjusted difference in PCHI associated with maternal asthma at birth was -0.77 (95% CI = -5.1, 3.5; p = 0.72).

Contrary to the initial hypothesis, maternal hypertension at birth was not associated with worse child PCHI at age 15 years. Among children whose mothers experienced no change in years of education between the child's birth and age 15 years, the adjusted difference in PCHI associated with maternal hypertension was -1.1 (95% CI = -3.5, 1.3; p = 0.4). Among mothers who completed additional years of education between their child's birth and age 15 years, the adjusted difference in PCHI associated with maternal asthma was -1.5 (95% CI = -2.8, -0.1; p = 0.05).

Discussion

The aim of this study was to identify whether a negative relationship existed between maternal health conditions at birth among ELGANs and positive child health, and whether this relationship could be moderated by SES factors. Maternal health conditions in both cases have a negative impact on PCHI but this impact is less significant and less dramatic when maternal education increases between birth and age 15 years.

There are several potential explanations for the findings of this study that require further investigation. For example, maternal obesity is associated with neonatal inflammation (15-17), and asthma has also been linked to inflammatory pathways in the placenta (18). Within the ELGAN cohort, there are previously reported associated between neonatal inflammation and adverse neurodevelopmental outcomes (16, 19). Mothers with an adverse health condition and a child with disabilities may be less likely to work outside the home, which could impact the socioeconomic level or healthcare quality of the child. The role of maternal education in moderating this relationship also needs to be explored. Among premature infants, socioeconomic disadvantage at birth has been associated with elevated neurobehavioral risks and poorer neurocognitive and academic outcomes at age 10 years (20, 21). Furthermore, maternal educational advancement during the child's first ten years of life is associated with modestly improved neurocognitive outcomes within the ELGAN cohort (21). This study indicates that maternal educational advancement during the child's first fifteen years of life could be associated with more positive child health.

Table 1. Comparison of ELGAN Study participants who were discharged alive from the neonatal intensive care unit, those evaluated at 10 years of age, and those evaluated at 15 years of age. Data are number of children (percent of group) (14)

Characteristics		Discharged Alive from NICU (n = 1222)	Age 10 (n = 889)	Age 15 (n = 694)
Maternal Age (years)	<21	174 (14)	115 (13)	80 (12)
	21-35	820 (67)	594 (67)	445 (67)
	>35	228 (19)	180 (20)	144 (22)
Unmarried Mother		533 (44)	353 (40)	235 (35)
Maternal Education (years)	≤12	521 (44)	367 (41)	250 (37)
	>12 to <16	276 (24)	210 (24)	153 (23)
	≥16	378 (32)	312 (35)	266 (40)
Mother Covered by Medicaid or Another State-supported Medical Insurance		483 (40)	314 (35)	217 (32)
Race	Asian, Native American, or mixed race	153 (13)	98 (11)	61 (9)
	Black	336 (28)	227 (26)	159 (24)
	White	722 (60)	562 (63)	449 (67)
Hispanic	Yes	147 (12)	86 (9.7)	57 (8.6)
	No	1068 (88)	800 (90)	609 (91)
Mother's Pre-pregnancy Body Mass Index (kg/m2)	<18.5	91 (7.8)	68 (7.9)	47 (7.3)
	18.5 to <30	824 (70)	595 (69)	444 (69)
	≥30	256 (22)	194 (23)	154 (24)
Cesarean Delivery		809 (66)	590 (66)	440 (66)

Table 1. (Continued)

Characteristics		Discharged Alive from NICU (n = 1222)	Age 10 (n = 889)	Age 15 (n = 694)
Sex	Male	638 (52)	455 (51)	341 (51)
	Female	584 (48)	434 (49)	328 (49)
Multiple gestation		365 (32)	293 (35)	236 (38)
Gestational Age (Weeks)	23-24	251 (21)	187 (21)	144 (22)
	25-26	562 (46)	400 (45)	305 (46)
	27	409 (34)	302 (34)	220 (33)
Birth Weight (Grams)	≤750	448 (37)	332 (37)	253 (38)
	750-1000	529 (43)	382 (43)	284 (43)
	>1000	245 (20)	175 (20)	132 (20)
Birth Weight Z-score < -2		65 (5.3)	53 (6.0)	41 (6.1)
Average Daily Weight Gain during neonatal intensive care	Lowest Quartile	301 (25)	207 (23)	156 (23)
	Highest Quartile	308 (25)	225 (25)	167 (25)
White Matter Injury on Neonatal Ultrasound		246 (20)	188 (21)	138 (21)
Chronic Lung Disease		616 (50)	461 (52)	357 (51)

Abbreviations: NICU – neonatal intensive care unit.

Table 2. Characteristics. Maternal and neonatal characteristics of participants grouped according to maternal health conditions at birth

Characteristics		Mother with asthma N = 200	Mother with pre-pregnancy diabetes N = 43	Mother with hypertension N = 312	Mother with obesity N = 323	Mother had none of those N = 829
Birth weight (g)	<= 750	83 (41.5%)	23 (53.5%)	186 (59.6%)	152 (47.1%)	336 (40.5%)
	751-1000	86 (43.0%)	15 (34.9%)	97 (31.1%)	126 (39.0%)	323 (39.0%)
	1001-1250	30 (15.0%)	1 (2.33%)	28 (8.97%)	42 (13.0%)	154 (18.6%)
	>1250	1 (0.50%)	4 (9.30%)	1 (0.32%)	3 (0.93%)	16 (1.93%)
Gestational age (weeks)	23-24	54 (27.0%)	11 (25.6%)	62 (19.9%)	90 (27.9%)	250 (30.2%)
	25-26	97 (48.5%)	13 (30.2%)	135 (43.3%)	145 (44.9%)	345 (41.6%)
	27	49 (24.5%)	19 (44.2%)	115 (36.9%)	88 (27.2%)	234 (28.2%)
Sex	Female	98 (49.0%)	19 (44.2%)	160 (51.3%)	152 (47.1%)	381 (46.0%)
	Male	102 (51.0%)	24 (55.8%)	152 (48.7%)	171 (52.9%)	448 (54.0%)
Mother's education (years)	<= 12	92 (46.0%)	18 (41.9%)	126 (40.4%)	146 (45.2%)	339 (40.9%)
	13-15	60 (30.0%)	13 (30.2%)	88 (28.2%)	106 (32.8%)	138 (16.6%)
	16+	45 (22.5%)	12 (27.9%)	83 (26.6%)	65 (20.1%)	267 (32.2%)
	Missing	3 (1.50%)	0 (0.00%)	15 (4.81%)	6 (1.86%)	85 (10.3%)
Medical insurance from Medicaid	No	104 (52.0%)	26 (60.5%)	177 (56.7%)	174 (53.9%)	468 (56.5%)
	Yes	96 (48.0%)	17 (39.5%)	125 (40.1%)	149 (46.1%)	300 (36.2%)
	Missing	0 (0.00%)	0 (0.00%)	10 (3.21%)	0 (0.00%)	61 (7.36%)
Bronchopulmonary dysplasia, O2 at 36 weeks	No	73 (36.5%)	12 (27.9%)	99 (31.7%)	116 (35.9%)	354 (42.7%)
	Yes	90 (45.0%)	25 (58.1%)	163 (52.2%)	141 (43.7%)	332 (40.0%)
	Missing	37 (18.5%)	6 (14.0%)	50 (16.0%)	66 (20.4%)	143 (17.2%)

Table 2. (Continued)

Characteristics		Mother with asthma N = 200	Mother with pre-pregnancy diabetes N = 43	Mother with hypertension N = 312	Mother with obesity N = 323	Mother had none of those N = 829
Brain white matter damage	No	153 (76.5%)	36 (83.7%)	274 (87.8%)	255 (78.9%)	667 (80.5%)
	Yes	41 (20.5%)	6 (14.0%)	35 (11.2%)	60 (18.6%)	128 (15.4%)
	Missing	6 (3.00%)	1 (2.33%)	3 (0.96%)	8 (2.48%)	34 (4.10%)
Birth weight (grams)		798 (187)	767 (257)	713 (194)	785 (194)	827 (202)
Birth weight z-score	< -2	10 (5.00%)	9 (20.9%)	71 (22.8%)	30 (9.29%)	26 (3.14%)
	< -1	33 (16.5%)	8 (18.6%)	90 (28.8%)	50 (15.5%)	82 (9.89%)
	< 0	72 (36.0%)	13 (30.2%)	86 (27.6%)	107 (33.1%)	334 (40.3%)
	>= 0	85 (42.5%)	13 (30.2%)	65 (20.8%)	136 (42.1%)	387 (46.7%)
Necrotizing enterocolitis	no/watch/I/II	185 (92.5%)	39 (90.7%)	276 (88.5%)	281 (87.0%)	750 (90.5%)
	Med	0 (0.00%)	0 (0.00%)	4 (1.28%)	3 (0.93%)	11 (1.33%)
	Surg	8 (4.00%)	4 (9.30%)	21 (6.73%)	24 (7.43%)	40 (4.83%)
	Perf	7 (3.50%)	0 (0.00%)	11 (3.53%)	14 (4.33%)	25 (3.02%)
	Missing	0 (0.00%)	0 (0.00%)	0 (0.00%)	1 (0.31%)	3 (0.36%)

Table 3. Outcomes. Age 15 years health outcomes of participants with follow-up data at age 15 years grouped according to maternal health conditions at birth.

Outcomes		Mother with asthma	Mother with pre-pregnancy diabetes	Mother with hypertension	Mother with obesity
PCHI Score	β (Unstratified)	-2.836 p = 0.0175	-4.6614 p = 0.0329	-0.8337 p = 0.4415	-3.671 p = 1.00E-04
	β (NO change in education)	-4.2891 p = 0.0048	-5.633 p = 0.0292	-1.0787 p = 0.4002	-4.6273 p = 1.00E-04
	β (+ change in education)	-0.7735 p = 0.7204	-3.7127 p = 0.435	-1.4532 p = .05126	-2.7143 p = 0.1525

This project breaks the cycle of children's health disparities by intervening where socioeconomic disparities link pregnancy vulnerability and physical health. This project is an attempt to break that connection with modifiable socioeconomic variables that can be addressed and/or mitigated by addressing socioeconomic disparities. Hopefully, it helps illustrate how changes in life over childhood may moderate adverse birth and health outcomes.

Furthermore, throughout the course of this study, the limitations of using change in maternal education as an indicator of socioeconomic status became apparent because this change is entirely one directional. Additionally, a positive change for this variable does not necessarily indicate an increase in quality of life, due to there being maximum values for education in the definition used by ELGAN investigators. Because this definition is hard to operationalize, we also intend to run regressions stratified according to average education, and to model the impacts of maternal education at birth and maternal education at age 15 years in separate analyses.

The most immediate next steps in this project are to use the same structure and strategy for other social determinants of health that were recorded both at birth and at follow up surveys, including public health insurance, single marital status, and food and nutritional service assistance. PCHI is analyzed as a continuous variable even though there is minimal gradation, so a more homogeneous continuous variable that could be used in this analysis is IQ. Additionally, 17-year data from the ELGAN study is being collected during this time, and it can be used to see if the associations between maternal health and children's health are still present at age 17 years like at ages 15 and 10 years. ELGAN investigators are also considering a more granular study that looks at the direct impact of discrimination on the health of individual children, but because of the rigidity of variables collected initially this study is a bit more difficult to design, but it has important implications for the effects of environmental health disparities on children's health. As shown in Figure 1, the bidirectional links between pregnancy vulnerability, socioeconomic disparities, and adverse health outcomes can be broken by an increase in maternal education. This effect is significant even after the birth of the child and is a clear example of breaking the cycle of children's health disparities because two of the health outcomes used to quantify positive child's health (asthma and obesity) were associated with poorer children's health outcomes when a mother had either of these conditions. However, these associations were significantly weakened when the mother's education level increased before the child turned 15 years of age. These results indicate that maternal education reduces the effects of maternal adverse health outcomes and is a successful mechanism to Break the Cycle of Children's Environmental Health Disparities.

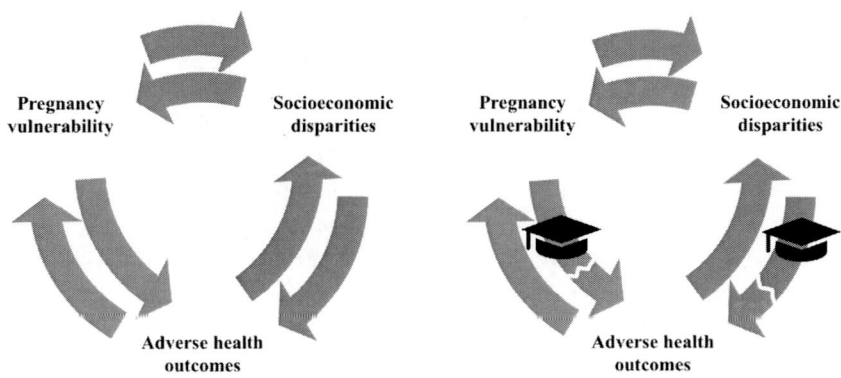

Figure 1. Breaking the cycle. Increasing maternal education between birth and age 15 years is associated with reduced adverse health effects among extremely low gestational age newborns.

Strengths and limitations

Strengths of the study are the large and diverse cohort originally recruited for the ELGAN study as well as the longitudinal data that has been collected for nearly the past 20 years. Other strengths of this prospective study include selection of participants based on gestational age rather than birth weight, which minimizes confounding related to fetal growth restriction. Finally, the rigorous training and protocol standardization procedures for recruitment and data collection resulted in high rates of complete data collection that allowed for integration of detailed measures of maternal, infant, and environmental characteristics.

A significant limitation of the study is the loss to follow up between birth and age 15 years and it is important to determine how the demographics of the follow-up subsets compare to the demographics of the original cohort in order to ascertain the generalizability of the study results and to investigate whether there are any common risk factors among those lost to follow-ups. Additionally, the rigidity of the variables that were collected initially makes it difficult to retroactively design studies that fully describe socioeconomic status in a multi-dimensional way.

Another limitation of this study is the fact that the data does not reflect current neonatal outcomes, because at the time of the study 23 weeks' gestation was typically the earliest an infant could survive, but now infants born at 22 weeks of gestation can survive. These less mature infants exhibit outcomes different from those described here, since gestational age is associated with a variety of health concerns regardless of socioeconomic status.

Finally, this study did not analyze gradation in educational changes; therefore, future studies should take into account how larger or smaller increases in education affect PCHI and whether there is a minimum level of educational change necessary to lessen the impact of maternal health conditions on positive child health.

Conclusion

This project evaluated the impact of socioeconomic status of mothers on health outcomes of their extremely low gestational age infants. Results indicated that maternal education can be used to break the link between adverse maternal health factors during pregnancy and adverse child health outcomes, or at least weaken this connection. The ELGAN study was not designed for environmental health investigations but for investigating inflammation and prematurity. However, this analysis has demonstrated that premature birth can be investigated from an environmental health perspective and that there is potential to break the cycle of children's environmental health disparities when using this lens.

Acknowledgments

Thank you to Dr Rebecca Fry, Dr T Michael O'Shea and Dr Kyle Roell. With gratitude to the Break the Cycle mentors, especially Dr Victoria Green. Finally, thank you to the children and their families who participated in this study, and to the ELGAN Study Investigators, listed below. Also acknowledge: Boston Children's Hospital, Boston MA: Janice Ware, Taryn Coster, Brandi Henson, Rachel Wilson, Kirsten McGhee, Patricia Lee, Aimee

Asgarian, Anjali Sadhwani. Tufts Medical Center, Boston MA: Ellen Perrin, Emily Neger, Kathryn Mattern, Jenifer Walkowiak, Susan Barron. University of Massachusetts Medical School, Worcester MA: Jean Frazier, Lauren Venuti, Beth Powers, Ann Foley, Brian Dessureau, Molly Wood, Jill Damon-Minow. Yale University School of Medicine, New Haven, CT: Richard Ehrenkranz, Jennifer Benjamin, Elaine Romano, Kathy Tsatsanis, Katarzyna Chawarska, Sophy Kim, Susan Dieterich, Karen Bearrs. Wake Forest University Baptist Medical Center, Winston-Salem NC: T Michael O'Shea, Nancy Peters, Patricia Brown, Emily Ansusinha, Ellen Waldrep, Jackie Friedman, Gail Hounshell, Debbie Allred. University Health Systems of Eastern Carolina, Greenville, NC: Stephen C Engelke, Nancy Darden-Saad, Gary Stainback. North Carolina Children's Hospital, Chapel Hill, NC: Diane Warner, Janice Wereszczak, Janice Bernhardt, Joni McKeeman, Echo Meyer. Helen DeVos Children's Hospital, Grand Rapids, MI: Steve Pastyrnak, Wendy Burdo-Hartman, Julie Rathbun, Sarah Nota, Teri Crumb. Sparrow Hospital, Lansing, MI: Madeleine Lenski, Deborah Weiland, Megan Lloyd. University of Chicago Medical Center, Chicago, IL: Scott Hunter, Michael Msall, Rugile Ramoskaite, Suzanne Wiggins, Krissy Washington, Ryan Martin, Barbara Prendergast, Megan Scott. William Beaumont Hospital, Royal Oak, MI: Judith Klarr, Beth Kring, Jennifer DeRidder, Kelly Vogt. Financial Support: This study was supported by the National Institute of Neurological Disorders and Stroke (5U01NS040069-09; 5U01NS04006-05), the National Institute of Child Health and Human Development (5P30HD018655-28), and the NIH ECHO Program (UG3OD023348-01).

References

[1] Bangma JT, Kwiatkowski E, Psioda M, Santos HP, Jr, Hooper SR, Douglass L, et al. Early life antecedents of positive child health among 10-year-old children born extremely preterm. Pediatr Res 2019;86(6):758-65.
[2] Bangma JT, Kwiatkowski E, Psioda M, Santos HP, Jr., Hooper SR, Douglass L, et al. Assessing positive child health among individuals born extremely preterm. J Pediatrics 2018;202:44-9.
[3] ElHassan NO, Bai S, Gibson N, Holland G, Robbins JM, Kaiser JR. The impact of prematurity and maternal socioeconomic status and education level on achievement-test scores up to 8th grade. PLoS One 2018;13(5):e0198083.
[4] Helderman JB, O'Shea TM, Kuban KC, Allred EN, Hecht JL, Dammann O, et al. Antenatal antecedents of cognitive impairment at 24 months in extremely low gestational age newborns. Pediatrics 2012;129(3):494-502.

[5] Kuban KC, Joseph RM, O'shea TM, Allred EN, Heeren T, Douglass L, et al. Girls and boys born before 28 weeks gestation: Risks of cognitive, behavioral, and neurologic outcomes at age 10 years. J Pediatrics 2016;173:69-75.

[6] Bright HR, Babata KB, Allred EN, Erdei C, Kuban KCK, Joseph RM, et al. Neurocognitive outcomes at 10 years of age in extremely preterm newborns with late-onset bacteremia. J Pediatrics 2017;187:43-9.

[7] Douglass LM, Heeren TC, Stafstrom CE, DeBassio W, Allred EN, Leviton A, et al. Cumulative incidence of seizures and epilepsy in ten-year-old children born before 28 weeks' gestation. Pediatr Neurol 2017;73:13-9.

[8] Rutter M, Bailey A, Lord C. The social communication questionnaire: Manual. Los Angeles, CA: Western Psychological Services, 2003.

[9] Le Couteur A, Lord C, Rutter M. The autism diagnostic interview-revised (ADI-R). Los Angeles, CA: Western Psychological Services, 2003.

[10] Joseph RM, O'Shea TM, Allred EN, Heeren T, Hirtz D, Paneth N, et al. Prevalence and associated features of autism spectrum disorder in extremely low gestational age newborns at age 10 years. Autism Res 2017;10(2):224-32.

[11] Scott MN, Hunter SJ, Joseph RM, O'Shea TM, Hooper SR, Allred EN, et al. Neurocognitive correlates of attention-deficit hyperactivity disorder symptoms in children born at extremely low gestational age. J Dev Behav Pediatr 2017;38(4):249-59.

[12] Gadow KD, Sprafkin J. Child symptom inventory 4: Screening and norms manual. Stony Brook, NY: Checkmate Plus, 2002.

[13] Sprafkin J, Gadow KD, Salisbury H, Schneider J, Loney J. Further evidence of reliability and validity of the Child Symptom Inventory-4: Parent checklist in clinically referred boys. J Clin Child Adolesc Psychol 2002;31(4):513-24.

[14] O'Shea TM, Register HM, Yi JX, Jensen ET, Joseph RM, Kuban K, et al. Growth during infancy after extremely preterm birth: Associations with later neurodevelopmental and health outcomes. J Pediatrics 2022:S0022-3476(22)00724-7.

[15] van der Burg JW, Sen S, Chomitz VR, Seidell JC, Leviton A, Dammann O. The role of systemic inflammation linking maternal BMI to neurodevelopment in children. Pediatr Res 2016;79(1-1):3-12.

[16] Kuban KC, O'Shea TM, Allred EN, Paneth N, Hirtz D, Fichorova RN, et al. Systemic inflammation and cerebral palsy risk in extremely preterm infants. J Child Neurol 2014;29(12):1692-8.

[17] van der Burg JW, Jensen ET, van de Bor M, Joseph RM, O'Shea TM, Kuban K, et al. Maternal obesity and attention-related symptoms in the preterm offspring. Early Hum Dev 2017;115:9-15.

[18] Meakin AS, Saif Z, Jones AR, Aviles PFV, Clifton VL. Review: Placental adaptations to the presence of maternal asthma during pregnancy. Placenta 2017;54:17-23.

[19] Allred EN, Dammann O, Fichorova RN, Hooper SR, Hunter SJ, Joseph RM, et al. Systemic inflammation during the first postnatal month and the risk of attention deficit hyperactivity disorder characteristics among 10 year-old children born extremely preterm. J Neuroimmune Pharmacol 2017;12(3):531-43.

[20] Hofheimer JA, Smith LM, McGowan EC, O'Shea TM, Carter BS, Neal CR, et al. Psychosocial and medical adversity associated with neonatal neurobehavior in infants born before 30 weeks gestation. Pediatr Res 2020;87(4):721-9.

[21] Joseph RM, O'Shea TM, Allred EN, Heeren T, Kuban KK. Maternal educational status at birth, maternal educational advancement, and neurocognitive outcomes at age 10 years among children born extremely preterm. Pediatr Res 2018;83(4):767-77.

Chapter 8

Factors that influence environmental health literacy from returning polycyclic aromatic hydrocarbon exposure results

Kylie W Riley[1,2], MPH
Kimberly Burke[1], MPH
Anabel Cole[1,2], MS, MPH
Maricela Ureno[1,2], MPH
Holly M Dixon[3], PhD
Lehyla Calero[1,2], MS
Lisa M Bramer[4], PhD
Katrina M Waters[3,4], PhD
Kim A Anderson[3], PhD
Julie B Herbstman[1,2,*], PhD, MSc
and Diana Rohlman[5], PhD

[1]Columbia Center for Children's Environmental Health, Columbia University, New York,
[2]Department of Environmental Health Sciences, Mailman School of Public Health, Columbia University, New York, United States of America
[3]Department of Environmental and Molecular Toxicology, Oregon State University, Corvallis, Oregon, United States of America
[4]Biological Sciences Division, Pacific Northwest National Labs, Richland, Washington
[5]School of Biological and Population Health Sciences, College of Public Health and Human Sciences, Corvallis, Oregon, United States of America

---

* *Correspondence:* Professor Julie Herbstman, Columbia University Mailman School of Public Health, 722 W168th Street, Room 1210, New York, NY 10032, United States. Email: jh2678@cumc.columbia.edu.

In: Environmental Health Disparities
Editors: I. Leslie Rubin and Joav Merrick
ISBN: 979-8-89113-487-4
© 2024 Nova Science Publishers, Inc.

Abstract

Reporting personal environmental exposure data back from researchers to study participants is becoming more common, however there are few tools to assess whether report back increases environmental health literacy (EHL). This study assessed whether sociodemographic or environmental characteristics were associated with changes in EHL after receiving personal air monitoring results. This study was conducted in a New York City based pregnancy cohort wherein participants were assessed for exposure to polycyclic aromatic hydrocarbons during the third trimester of pregnancy. Participants (n = 168) received their results two to five years after participation and a subset (n = 47) completed a survey evaluating perspectives on their results and subsequent behaviors. Using these results, we created a quantitative scale of EHL, with higher scores indicative of higher EHL. We found that participants with a college degree were significantly more likely to be surprised by their results than those with less than a high school degree (OR = 5.60, p ≤ 0.05) and that higher naphthalene levels were associated with decreased odds of being surprised about receiving the results (OR = 0.37, p = 0.02). There were no observed associations between demographic or exposure characteristics and our dichotomous EHL indicator; however, those with more education and higher income tended to have higher EHL scores. Additionally, participants who reported being surprised by or glad to receive their results had higher EHL scores. Open-ended text responses indicated that while some participants felt worried after receiving their results, participants reported being glad to have received the report.

Introduction

Environmental health literacy (EHL) is an emerging field that combines elements from different disciplines, including health literacy, risk communication, environmental health, communications research, and safety culture (1, 2). Building on the concept of health literacy (3), as EHL increases, it is anticipated that informed individuals can take control of their own health and be aware of how their actions may reduce exposure or mitigate risk from environmental hazards (1,2). These are valuable skills to have in a culture that is more aware of environmental exposures and changes including climate change (4). One potential route to increase EHL is through personal exposure report back (5-8).

Personal exposure report back is intended to return a research participant's own data and provide information about their study results. Previously, it was commonplace to return results to participants only if there was clinical guidance on the exposure levels (5). However, in the last two decades, there has been a shift towards giving participants the option to receive their results back, even in the absence of a clinical cut point (5,9,10). To give guidance on how best to report back personal exposure monitoring, the Silent Spring Institute developed a handbook on report back (11). It includes sections on how to get started, methods for reporting back both environmental monitoring and biomonitoring results, and evaluation of the report back. With the ethical shift regarding research participants' right to know and a handbook on best practices, reporting back results has become more commonplace, and is now recommended (9).

At the most basic level, the return of personal results addresses a commitment to scientific transparency, as it also addresses a core element of EHL: recognition of environmental exposures. Finn and O'Fallon adapted Bloom's taxonomy of educational objectives to environmental health knowledge, which outlines gradual steps of increased literacy around environmental health issues with concepts including recognition, understanding, application, analysis, evaluation, and creation (2). While the EHL taxonomy is a useful framework for demonstrating how individuals learn and progress in EHL, it does not provide an indicator to measure EHL.

To date, there have been few tools developed to assess EHL. Studies have looked at qualitative changes associated with return of data and seen increases (6-8), but quantitative measures are less common. Some of the current methods to measure EHL rely on concepts from health literacy, which is not necessarily the same as EHL (12-14). Our goal in this study was to determine whether sociodemographic or environmental characteristics were associated with both quantitative and qualitative changes in EHL among research participants after receiving report back on personal results.

In this study we look at a New York City based pregnancy cohort with personal chemical exposure monitoring conducted for polycyclic aromatic hydrocarbons (PAH) in the third trimester of pregnancy. The cohort comes from an urban area, is primarily Hispanic, and is often an understudied research population. Participants received their personal results back between two and five years after the monitoring was conducted. The time between participation and return of results was included as a potential predictive variable. The motivating factor for this research is to find a way to break the cycle of children's environmental health disparities, utilizing report back to increase recognition and understanding of how environmental exposures impact health.

Our study

Pregnant individuals enrolled in the Fair Start cohort of the Columbia Center for Children's Environmental Health (CCCEH) participated in this study. Recruitment of the Fair Start cohort began in 2013 at New York Presbyterian Ambulatory Care clinics in New York City. The cohort was established with the goal of characterizing the association between prenatal and early life environmental exposures on childhood development. Recruitment into the Fair Start Cohort remains ongoing, with a planned sample size of at least 750 participants. This study was conducted with a subset of participants that were enrolled between November 2015 through March 2019. Participants primarily reside in the neighborhoods of Northern Manhattan and the South Bronx and 90% self-identify as Hispanic, as previously described (15). As part of participation in the cohort, individuals completed prenatal visits during the third trimester of pregnancy, which included completing questionnaires to collect information on demographics, occupation, environmental exposures, and personal product use. Following the prenatal visit, participants wore a passive sampling silicone wristband for 48 hours, to assess their personal exposure to semi-volatile and volatile organic compounds. The wristbands were analyzed at Oregon State University for 63 PAHs.

Return of data to study participants development

Personalized reports were created for a total of 168 participants summarizing their PAH exposure, as measured by the wristbands. The report included a personalized cover letter, infographics summarizing how PAHs are generated, where they are found and ways to reduce PAH exposure. Though the wristbands measured 63 PAHs, and all data was returned, the reports focused on n = 18 PAHs, which have been identified as priority chemicals by the United States Environmental Protection Agency (EPA) and the Agency for Toxic Substances and Disease Registry (ATSDR). The EPA identifies 16 PAHs as priority PAHs, operating under the rationale that these 16 are representative of environmental exposures, although this assumption has been questioned (16). The ATSDR highlighted PAHs as a chemical group on their Priority Substance list (17), with the toxicological profile for PAHs identifying 17 specific PAHs (18). These 17 PAHs were selected based on the availability of health and toxicity data, probability of human exposure, and potential for adverse health outcomes following exposure (18). When the EPA and ATSDR lists are combined, there are 18 unique PAHs.

Individual plots were generated comparing each person's individual exposure to naphthalene and phenanthrene, which are two priority PAH that were selected, as they were the most commonly detected PAHs in the wristbands; both were detected in >75% of samples. Plots compared each participant to the other participants in the study. Each report also included a personalized table showing which of the priority PAHs were detected along with common environmental sources of these chemicals, the total number of PAHs detected in the individual's wristband, and a table detailing the concentration of each PAH found in the individual's wristband and the range of exposure across the study population.

This report was based on a previously developed report (9), then piloted and tested in focus groups within the cohort. Feedback and revisions from the focus group were incorporated prior to utilizing the report with the participants for this study (Riley et al, manuscript in preparation). Reports were generated in English and in Spanish, and paper copies were sent to the participants' homes in June 2021, with electronic versions emailed upon request. A short (04:48 min) video (19) was developed to walk participants through the report, with English and Spanish closed captioning. This study was approved by the Columbia University Irving Medical Center IRB (#AAAK6753) and Oregon State University IRB (IRB-2021-1048) and individuals were consented prior to their prenatal visit.

Survey

Following receipt of the results in July of 2021, participants (n = 168) were sent a link to an electronic survey to gather feedback on the report using the REDCap system of the Data Coordinating Center at the Mailman School of Public Health, Columbia University. The survey was available in both English and Spanish, with the option for participants to select the language they were fluent in. All individuals who received a report were eligible to complete the survey, which consisted of 18 questions regarding socio-demographics, report readability, time spent reviewing the report, level of interest in receiving their results, and whether the participants were surprised by the results. Survey questions were chosen to assess environmental health literacy, and included questions adapted from the Silent Spring Institute Report Back Handbook (11). The survey questions are included in the *supplemental material*. A total of N = 47 participants completed the questionnaire, resulting in a 28% completion rate. Prior to analysis, open ended questions with responses in Spanish were translated into English by a native Spanish speaker.

Table 1. Demographic characteristics and exposure summaries of participants included in the research study[a]

Level	No Survey	Completed Survey	p-value
N	121	47	
Maternal Age (mean (SD))	28.96 (6.43)	28.71 (5.25)	0.82
Categorical Characteristics[b]			
Maternal Education (%)			
<High School	23 (20.9)	12 (26.7)	0.50
High School Diploma	48 (43.6)	15 (33.3)	
2- or 4-Year College Degree	39 (35.5)	18 (40)	
Marital Status			
Never Married	56 (50.9)	17 (37.8)	0.20
Married/Living with Partner	48 (43.6)	23 (51.1)	
Divorced/Separated	6 (5.5)	5 (11.1)	
Income			
$0-$20,000	58 (52.7)	29 (64.4)	0.25
>$20,000	52 (47.3)	16 (35.6)	
Ethnicity			
Hispanic or Latino	105 (95.5)	45 (100.0)	0.34
Not Hispanic or Latino	5 (4.5)	0 (0.0)	
PAH Exposure			
Naphthalene[c] (mean (SD))	4.54 (0.89)	4.57 (1.19)	0.84
Phenanthrene[c] (mean (SD))	5.61 (0.61)	5.67 (0.50)	0.62
Total PAH Count[d] (mean (SD))	11.49 (4.52)	11.09 (5.59)	0.63
Count of Priority PAH[e] (mean (SD))	5.01 (2.14)	4.38 (2.33)	0.10

[a]Utilized Fisher's Exact test for comparisons.
[b]Categorical characteristic data is only available for 155 participants (data were unavailable for 13 participants).
[c]Unit = log pmol/wristband.
[d]Total number of PAH found in wristband, wristbands were analyzed for 63 PAHs.
[e]The PAH method includes 18 Priority PAHs, as defined by ATSDR and the EPA.

Development of the EHL scale

We developed a numeric scale to assess EHL based on the information collected in the survey. First, we selected appropriate questions from the survey based on their applicability to the EHL taxonomy (2). A total EHL indicator was created by selecting Likert questions from the survey that were associated with different levels of the EHL framework (2). Table 1 includes a full list of questions used, which include a measure of participant likelihood to change behavior in response to exposures, a key tenet of EHL (2,20). Responses to each of these questions were categorized and coded based on Likert responses—where higher numbers indicate higher EHL. Scores for each question were summed to create an EHL scale with a minimum of 0 and a maximum possible score of 26. The median value was 14 (range 8-20).

Text mining

Data was collected for 47 participants. A total of 33 participants answered the question "What are your feelings after viewing your results?". Standard text processing steps were taken to convert to lower case text, remove punctuation, remove standard English stop words using the Snowball stemmer project (21), and remove white space. A sentiment analysis (22) was conducted on each participant's answer. The presence of words corresponding to 6 different emotions ("anticipation," "fear," "joy," "sadness," "surprise," "trust") was tabulated along with the overall sentiment ("negative," "positive"). A predicted probability was calculated for the sentiments: positive, negative, and neutral. For each participant, the predicted sentiment was taken to be the sentiment with the highest respective probability.

Data analysis

To determine the representativeness of those who completed the survey versus those who did not, we used Fisher's exact test to account for the small sample size. Quantitative data analysis focused on potentially modifiable factors that influenced how participants perceived their report back information. Child age at report (as a proxy for time between exposure monitoring and receipt of report), maternal education, marital status, and income were all examined as predictors in the analysis.

Exposure to naphthalene and phenanthrene were also considered as potentially modifiable factors that might be associated with EHL. Given the high detection frequency, these two chemicals were specifically highlighted in the report and more detail was provided about them for the benefit of the participants. Values were log adjusted and treated as predictors in the models. Additionally, we evaluated the total number of PAHs detected and the number of priority PAHs found in each person's wristband as predictors of exposure.

Linear and logistic regression models were used, as appropriate, to assess whether the potentially modifiable lifestyle and exposure factors listed above were associated with indicators of EHL. *Supplementary Table 1* summarizes the development and scoring of the variable. In addition to multivariate models, we also compared the reaction to the results (e.g., surprised, glad) by EHL score using t-tests. All analyses were completed in R statistical software (R version 4.1.2) (18).

A thematic analysis was conducted on participant responses to the question "What were your feelings after viewing the results?" Each response was manually reviewed and coded. Three themes were identified: worried, reassured, and wanting to learn more. One respondent noted not having any feelings after the return of results, and their answers were excluded from this analysis.

Findings

Participants who completed the survey (n = 47) were not statistically different from participants who received their report but did not complete the survey with respect to maternal age, education, marital status, income, ethnicity, and PAH exposure. While not statistically significant, participants who completed the survey were more likely (p = 0.20) to be married or living with their partner for >7 years than participants who did not complete the survey (see Table 2).

Table 2. Average environmental health literacy score by demographic characteristics

Level	Average EHL Score Mean (SD)	p-value
N = 44		
Maternal Education (%)		
<High School	14.70 (3.33)	0.56
High School Diploma	15.86 (2.85)	0.10
2 or 4 Year College Degree	16.94 (2.13)	0.50

Level	Average EHL Score Mean (SD)	p-value
N = 44		
Marital Status		
Never Married	15.67 (2.99)	
Married/ Living with Partner	16.14 (2.85)	0.63
Divorced/ Separated	17.00 (1.63)	
Income		
$0-$20,000	15.62 (2.91)	0.19
>$20,000	16.75 (2.46)	
Ethnicity		
Hispanic or Latino	16.05 (2.78)	
Not Hispanic or Latino	N/A	

General response to the report

Respondents were asked simple questions to gauge their response to the report. Specifically, participants were asked if they were glad to have received their results, and if they were surprised by their results. N = 47 participants (28% of the study population who received their reports) responded to these questions, and a majority were glad to have received their data (94%) and were surprised by any of their results (69%).

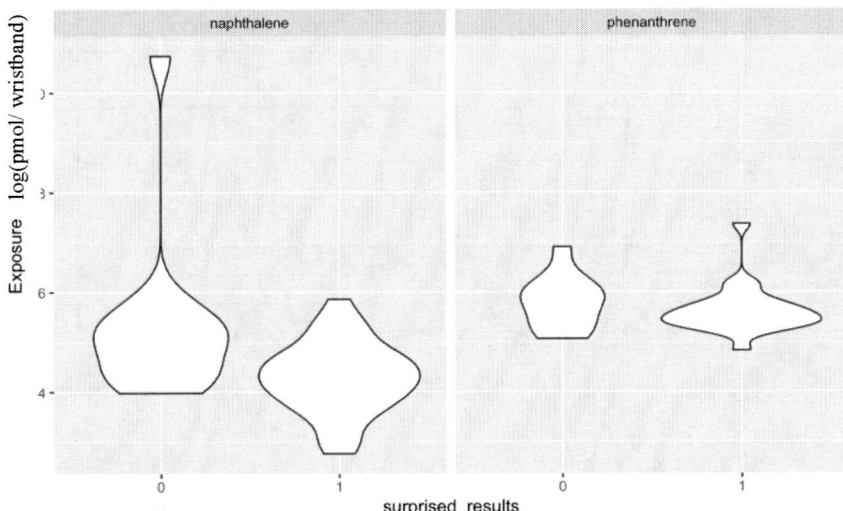

Figure 1. Distribution of naphthalene and phenanthrene by participant response to whether they were surprised by their results.

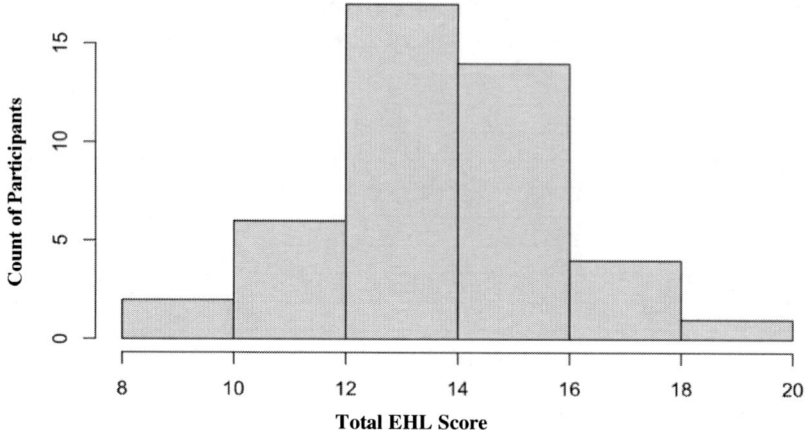

Figure 2. Distribution of environmental health literacy (EHL) indicator score. Maximum possible score = X. Scores ranged from 8-20.

Table 3. Summary of model summary data

	Surprised Results[1]		Glad to have learned Results[1]		Time Reading[2]		Total EHL Score[2]	
Outcome	OR	P Value	OR	P Value	OR	P value	Beta	P Value
Child Age	1.59	0.27	1.24	0.78	0.77	0.59	-0.11	0.83
Maternal Education								
High school diploma	3.30	0.16	1.27	0.87	4.67	0.21	0.08	0.48
2- or 4-year degree	5.60	0.05*	1.55	0.77	1.67	0.58	0.14	0.16
Marital Status	1.04	0.96	2.93	0.40	3.23	0.21	0.47	0.63
Income	1.30	0.71	17.41	0.99	0.69	0.66	0.07	0.37
Naphthalene	0.37	0.02*	0.87	0.72	1.03	0.94	-0.85	0.02*
Phenanthrene	1.88	0.31	22.08	0.24	1.43	0.80	-0.65	0.49
Total PAH	1.01	0.37	1.03	0.12	1.15	0.14	-0.002	0.97
Priority PAH	0.90	0.48	0.94	0.26	1.27	0.18	-0.16	0.37

*Indicates significance at a level of $p < 0.05$.
[1] logistic regression model.
[2] linear regression model.

We found that mothers with a college degree were significantly more likely to be surprised by their results than mothers with less than a high school degree (OR = 5.60, $p \leq 0.05$). We did not observe that income, marital status, and child age was associated with participants being surprised by their report, whether they were glad to have received their report, or the amount of time spent reading their report (see Table 3).

We observed that naphthalene levels were associated with a decreased odds of being surprised about receiving the results (OR = 0.37, p = 0.02) (see Figure 1). Phenanthrene, total number of PAHs detected, and the number of priority PAHs detected were not associated with being surprised by the report, being glad to have received the results, or time spent reading the report (see Table 3).

Environmental health literacy

A total of 44 participants (94% of all who completed the survey) answered all the questions used to create the EHL indicator score. The highest possible EHL score was 26. Scores ranged from 8-20, with a mean and median of 14 (see Figure 2). When examining EHL score by demographic characteristics, EHL score increased with increasing education, marital status, and income, although these trends were not statistically significant (see Table 2). When looking at measures of PAH exposure, naphthalene has an inverse association with total EHL score (β = -0.85, p = 0.02). Phenanthrene, total PAH, and priority PAH count were not associated with total EHL score (see Table 3). We observed that those who reported being surprised by their results had higher EHL scores than those who were not surprised (mean EHL = 17.2 (SD = 1.9) vs. 13.9 (SD = 2.9), p < 0.01) and those who were glad to receive their results had higher EHL scores than those who were not glad (mean EHL = 16.5 (SD = 2.4) vs. 11.3 (SD = 3.5), p < 0.01) (models not shown).

Reception of the report back

A total of 33 participants (70% of those who completed the survey) provided free-form responses to the question, "What are your feelings after viewing your results?" Responses in Spanish were translated to English. Open-text responses ranged from one word to 23 words, with a median word count of three words. The responses are visualized in supplemental Figure 1.

A sentiment analysis was conducted to evaluate the overall feelings reported by the participants. Words associated with six different emotions were characterized, with the most prevalent emotion being associated with the response being characterized as fear, followed by surprise, and then joy and anticipation (see Figure 3). The responses were further assessed for overall predicted sentiment (negative, neutral, positive). There were equal numbers of positive and negative associations, with slightly more responses being identified as neutral (see Figure 4).

Thematic analysis of the short answers resulted in three shared themes: wanting to learn more; being worried, and feeling reassured. There were six responses that referenced wanting to know more about their exposures. For example, one participant wrote: "I want to know more because I already know that I do not know anything about my exposures."

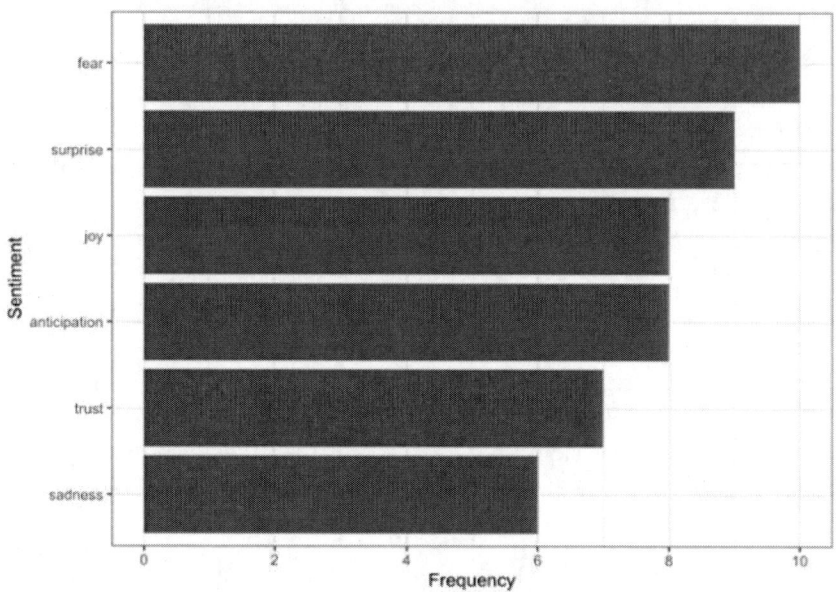

Figure 3. Total number of words corresponding to one of six emotions ("anticipation," "fear," "joy," "sadness," "surprise," "trust") across 33 open-ended responses in answer to the question, "What are your feelings after viewing your results?".

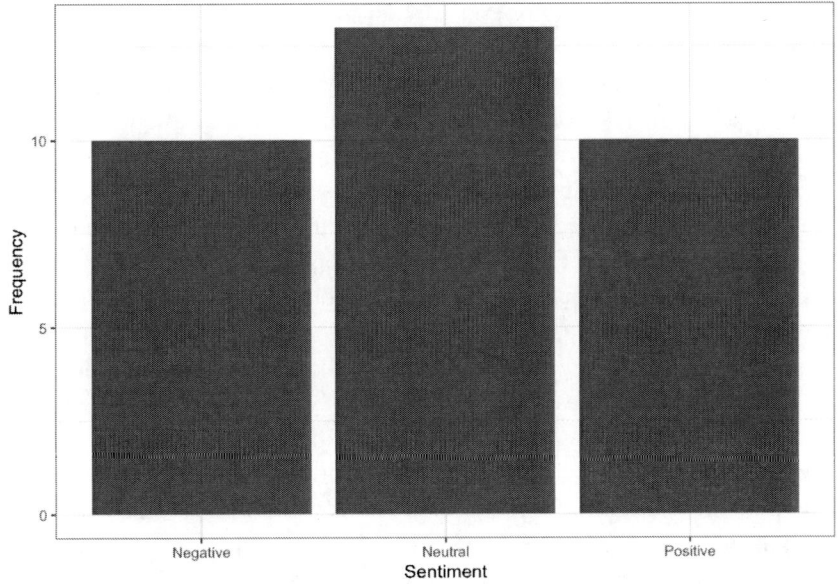

Figure 4. Frequency of predicted sentiments for 33 open-ended responses in answer to the question, "What are your feelings after viewing your results?"

The majority of responses (n = 16) were coded as indicating worry, with responses either directly using the word "worry" or obliquely referencing worry, as indicated by this participant: "Second thinking what items I surround myself with."

There were also several participants that referenced a feeling of reassurance (n = 8). As one respondent wrote, "Feeling more tranquility and gratitude for the information."

Discussion

The role of report-back is posited to help increase EHL, thereby facilitating individual knowledge gain and potential behavior changes (20,23,24). We returned individual data within the context of the study population to 168 individuals in the Fair Start Cohort, approximately 2-5 years after data collection. Over one-quarter of the participants completed a survey describing their reaction to the report. The survey respondent population was representative of the study population when assessed across sociodemographic variables.

Here, our data indicates that participants who are more educated (college degree +) and those with lower environmental exposures to common PAHs are more likely to be surprised by their results. Being surprised about receiving personal exposure monitoring information is indicative of being able to Recognize and Understand environmental health concepts, based on the EHL taxonomy by Finn and O'Fallon (2). In the taxonomy, the ability to Recognize and Understand a concept are at the most basic levels of EHL. An individual could progress through higher levels that include being able to Apply, Analyze, Evaluate, and eventually Create. College educated individuals may have been exposed to these concepts previously or be able to apply them to their daily life more easily. However, the question was binary (yes/no) and did not allow us to query the direction of surprise, (e.g., we do not know whether the participants were surprised that their levels were higher versus lower than they expected).

The negative association between naphthalene exposure and being surprised by the results is noteworthy and was unchanged after accounting for income and/or education. Naphthalene is a common air pollutant that is formed through several sources leading to exposure in ambient air including gasoline and oil combustion, as well as biomass burning, but also has several indoor exposure sources including mothballs, plug-in air fresheners, fumigants, and deodorizers (19). Individuals may be more familiar with these indoor sources of PAH, and naphthalene has a characteristic 'chemical' smell.

Beyond assessing the impact of individual return of results on participant reaction to the reports, we developed a measure of EHL using survey questions. There are few tools for measuring EHL (12-14, 24-26). Given the distribution, we did not set parameters of high versus low literacy like other tools (11, 21) yet looked at EHL as a continuous variable. We saw a positive trend between maternal education and EHL, although this relationship was not statistically significant, possibly due to the small sample size. Some tools have found significant associations between EHL and education (13), yet this has not been replicated in other EHL tools (14,27). We may have not seen this in our data because of the small sample size (n = 44) or because the categories chosen to group the data were slightly skewed with a smaller proportion of mothers not completing high school. Additionally, education status alone may not be the driver of EHL, compared to topic-specific knowledge. For example, a study looking at specific environmental exposures found that one component of EHL "willingness to engage in protective behaviors" was significantly associated with knowledge of the exposure as opposed to general educational attainment (27), yet in another study, content-specific knowledge was not associated with health-protective behaviors (13). In our study, we did not assess knowledge about PAH exposure explicitly so could not assess whether our indicator of education represents the contribution of educational attainment or knowledge specifically about PAH.

We saw that people were glad to have received the report, despite having participated in the research two to five years prior. The use of text mining for semantic analysis indicated equivalent negative and positive feelings across six emotions. Another study evaluated eight feelings ("curious," "Informed," "Interested," "Empowered," "Respected," "Helpless," "Scared," and "Worried") across a cohort of 295 women viewing results from blood tests, which included levels of flame retardants, PFAS, and lipids (28). Following structured interviews, most participants reported positive feelings before and after viewing their results, with a minority of participants reporting feeling helpless, scared, or worried (28). However, the authors noted that a more stratified analysis by race showed that the level of worry may differ by race, although this was complicated by the chemical results, as Black participants had higher levels of chemicals and noted higher levels of worry (28). Our cohort predominantly identified as Hispanic or Latino, and thus stratification of results by race was not possible. Beyond the semantic analysis, our qualitative analysis indicated that while participant responses referenced "worry," they also identified potential behavior changes, i.e., selecting different products to reduce exposures. Unfortunately, our survey characterized "worry" on a binary scale (yes/no) and did not allow for a more nuanced understanding.

Despite referencing fear upon viewing the results, participants overwhelmingly reported they were glad to have received their data (94%). In addition, eight of 30 responses expressed reassurance and gratitude for the report. This is borne out by other studies that have returned individual results, wherein participants were glad they had received their data (5,8,29-32). In particular, this is supported by prior data, wherein parents received information on children's exposures to asthma triggers (32). Participants in low income, public housing with lower socioeconomic status, similar to our cohort, found that the return of data was positively received and there was evidence that the reports facilitated greater understanding of environmental exposures (32). Here, our cohort is somewhat homogenous when looking at socioeconomic status, and thus we were not able to probe connections between socioeconomic status and EHL. Of note, the link between socioeconomic status and EHL has been found to be null in a study evaluating EHL levels and connections to adoption of health protective behaviors (27).

EHL is a complex concept that merges background information on environmental health, risk communication, public health, and behavioral science (6). The complex interplay between demographics, foundational environmental health knowledge, and perceptions of self-efficacy/knowledge sufficiency has been previously explored (14, 27). We were unable to probe into self-efficacy and knowledge sufficiency in this research; our survey included one question regarding likelihood to make changes (supplemental material: Questionnaire, Q8), yet was not designed to probe knowledge sufficiency as a co-variate for EHL, and thus was integrated into the overall measure rather than a standalone metric. While this data supports continued efforts to return individual data, the null associations between EHL and sociodemographic variables, as well as exposure predictors, suggest we need to better understand predictors of EHL to ensure reports are appropriate. It is frequently assumed that EHL and health literacy are similar, so the same predictors will apply to both concepts, but preliminary research suggests the relationship is more complicated (27). Indicators of health literacy include demographics such as age, gender, and marital status (33). When thinking about developing report back tools, we need to determine drivers specifically of EHL, rather than assuming drivers of health literacy.

Strengths of this study include conducting the report back in a longitudinal cohort study where participants remain engaged many years following data collection. CCCEH partnered with collaborators at Oregon State University who have previous experience returning results (8,34), to generate a report that was meaningful and culturally sensitive. Additionally, the version of the report that was used in this study had previously been piloted in the Fair Start cohort and undergone focus group feedback to improve the readability. Limitations of this research include having a small sample size (n = 47 completed the survey, n = 44 had all questions answered for EHL indicator variable). While the sample was representative of the larger cohort, more respondents may have allowed identification of predictors of EHL. Additionally, this data is collected in a primarily Hispanic urban cohort, and the generalizability of these results may not be applicable to other groups or locations.

This works helps to Break the Cycle of environmental health disparities by breaking the link between limited education/limited empowerment, thus leading to increased exposure then to negative health outcomes (see Figure 5). Reporting back data, following established ethical guidelines (5, 9, 30, 35), can increase EHL (6-8). Increased EHL is tied to increased knowledge, either general (12, 13) or topic-specific (27), leading to increased willingness to engage in behaviors to reduce exposure (27, 30, 32). In this way, the link leading to increased exposure is broken. Within the larger Fair Start cohort, previous work has shown that participants used information from their report to make informed decisions about reducing exposures, and became vocal in their community to raise awareness about environmental exposures (36). This is shown in other studies, wherein return of results can lead to behavior change, or willingness to change behavior, to reduce exposures and improve health (30, 32).

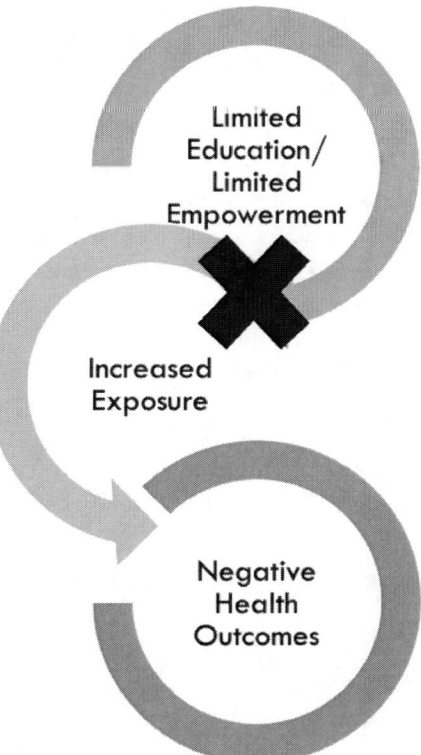

Figure 5. Cycle diagram.

Acknowledgments

This research was funded by the National Institutes of Environmental Health Sciences: grant numbers P30 ES030287 (Oregon State University Pacific Northwest Center for Translational Environmental Health Research), NIEHS R33 ES024718, and National Institutes of Health: grant number UH3 OD023290. Pacific Northwest National Laboratory is a multi-program laboratory operated by Battelle for the U.S. Department of Energy under Contract DE-AC05-76RL01830. We would like to thank Leslie Rubin and all of the Break the Cycle Faculty and Staff for their guidance and support. We would like to thank the Fair Start Cohort team for their work in data collection. Last, but certainly not least, thank you to the Fair Start participants for their continued participation and engagement with the study. Conflict of interest statement: Kim A. Anderson and Diana Rohlman, authors of this research, discloses a financial interest in MyExposome, Inc., which is marketing products (wristbands) related to the research being reported. The terms of this arrangement have been reviewed and approved by Oregon State University in accordance with its policy on research conflicts of interest. The authors have no other disclosures.

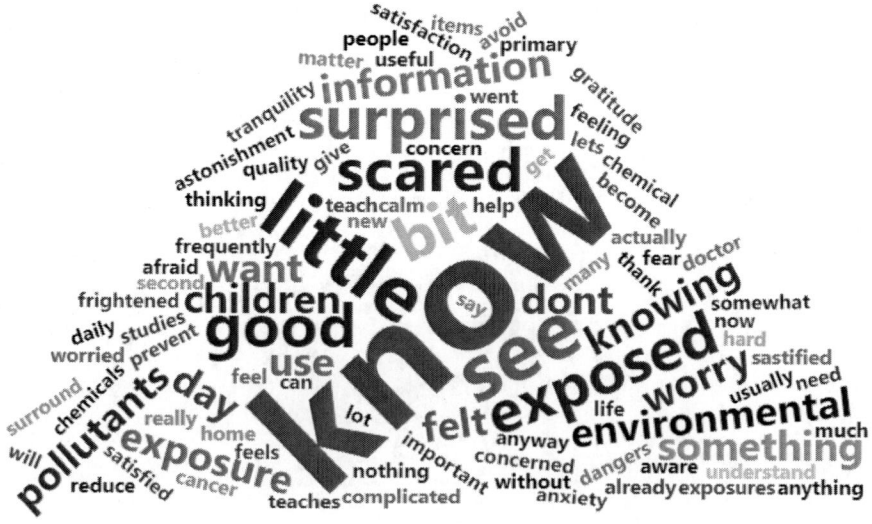

Supplemental Figure 1. Word cloud of words seen in open-ended question, "What are your feelings after viewing your results?"

Supplemental material

Questions from the report back questionnaire

The survey included some questions from the *Handbook for Reporting Results to Participants in Biomonitoring and Personal Exposure Studies* and are marked with an asterisk* or a double asterisk** if adapted.
- Dunagan SC, Brody JG, Morello-Frosch R, Brown P, Goho S, Tovar J, Patton S, Danford R. When Pollution is Personal: Handbook for Reporting Results to Participants in Biomonitoring and Personal Exposure Studies. Appendix E. California Household Exposure Study Interview. Silent Spring Institute; 2013.

1. How long did you spend reading your report?
    a. Less than 5 minutes
    b. 5-15 minutes
    c. More than 15 minutes
    d. I did not read it
2. What information were you MOST interested in reading about in the newsletter?
    a. Page 1 introductory letter
    b. Information about PAHs (human health, sources)
    c. Reducing exposure to PAHs
    d. Type of PAHs found in your wristband
    e. Your results
    f. The results of the whole study
3. How easy or hard to read and understand was each part of the report? (very easy, somewhat easy, neutral, difficult, very difficult, did not read)
    a. Page 1 introductory letter
    b. Information about PAHs (human health, sources)
    c. Reducing exposure to PAHs
    d. Type of PAHs found in your wristband
    e. Your results
    f. The results of the whole study
4. Before you received this report how much did you know about PAHs and the risk they pose to people?
    a. I knew a lot about PAHs

b. I knew a little about PAHs
c. I did not know anything about PAHs
5. How much did this report add to your knowledge about PAHs?
   a. A lot
   b. A moderate amount
   c. A little
   d. None at all
6. How easy or difficult was it for you to find what YOUR levels of PAHs were?
   a. Very easy
   b. Easy
   c. Neutral
   d. Difficult
   e. Very difficult
   f. I did not find this information
   g. I did not read the report
7. How easy or difficult was it for you to figure out how YOUR levels of PAHs compared to the whole group?
   a. Very easy
   b. Easy
   c. Neutral
   d. Difficult
   e. Very difficult
   f. I did not find this information
   g. I did not read the report
8. Which of the suggested steps to reduce PAH exposures are you most likely to take?
   a. Ventilate when cooking or using a wood-fired stove/fire (run fans or open windows). Grill or smoke outdoors.
   b. Limit exposure to gasoline and diesel fumes
   c. Replace pest control methods like mothballs with alternatives like cedar shavings
   d. Avoid e-cigarettes and cigarette/cigar smoke
   e. Rotate smoked, grilled and charbroiled foods with baked, steamed, and/or canned foods
   f. If you use a wood stove, make sure the opening and chimney do not leak smoke
   g. I am going to do something else:
   h. Other

Factors that influence environmental health literacy ... 157

    i. I am not going to do any of these things

9. Do you plan to talk about this study and/or your PAH exposure with a doctor, nurse, or public health professional?**
   a. I definitely will
   b. I probably will not
   c. I may or may not
   d. I probably will not
   e. I definitely will not
10. Please tell us a little about your experience receiving your study results. Was the report helpful to you, and are you glad you received this information about PAHs and the levels of PAHs we found in the wristbands you wore?
11. Did the description of how to read your results (see example graph) help you better understand your results? (1 = not easy, 10 = very easy)

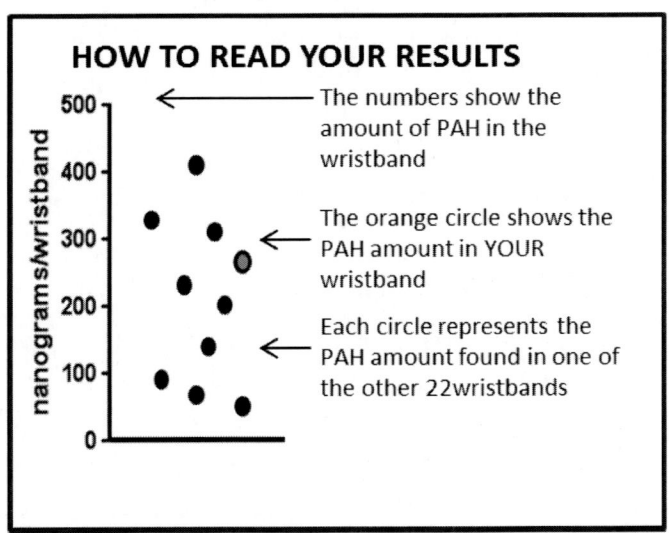

12. Overall, how interesting was it to see your chemical exposure results? (1 = not interesting, 10 = very interesting)
13. Are you glad to have learned about your own results?* (yes/no)
14. What are your feelings after viewing your results?**
15. Were you surprised by anything in the results? What was surprising?*
16. Did the study change your views about what role you think chemicals might play in your health?**

17. What additional resources or information would you like to have as a result of this study?*

Supplemental Table 1. Coding for the environmental health literacy indicator variable

Survey Question	Corresponding EHL Taxonomy	Scoring Summary
How long did you spend reading the report?	General EHL indicator	1 = Less than 5 minutes 2 = 5-15 minutes 3 = More than 15 minutes 0 = I did not read it
Before you received this report how much did you know about PAHs and the risk they pose to people?	Recognize	2 = I knew a lot about PAHs 1 = I knew a little about PAHs 0 = I did not know anything about PAHs
How much did this report add to your knowledge about PAHs?	Apply	3 = A lot 2 = A moderate amount 1 = A little 0 = None at all
How easy or difficult was it for you to find what YOUR levels of PAHs were?	Understand	3 = Easy 2 = Neutral 1 = Difficult 0 = I did not find this information 0 = I did not read the report
How easy or difficult was it for you to figure out how YOUR levels of PAHs compared to the whole group?	Understand	3 = Easy 2 = Neutral 1 = Difficult 0 = I did not find this information 0 = I did not read the report
Which of the suggested steps to reduce PAH exposures are you most likely to take?	Analyze	Sum of 8 options (range 0-8)
Do you plan to talk about this study and/or your PAH exposure with a doctor, nurse, or public health professional?	Evaluate	4 = I definitely will 3 = I probably will not 2 = I may or may not 1 = I probably will not 0 = I definitely will not

Survey questions were coded to the EHL taxonomy, described by Finn and O'Fallon (Finn, S. and O'Fallon, L., 2017. The emergence of environmental health literacy—from its roots to its future potential. Environmental health perspectives, 125(4), pp. 495-501.)

References

[1] Lindsey M, Chen S-R, Ben R, Manoogian M, Spradlin J. Defining environmental health literacy. Int J Environ Res Public Health 2021;18(21):11626.

[2] Finn S, O'Fallon L. The emergence of environmental health literacy—from its roots to its future potential. Environ Health Perspect 2017;125(4):495-501.

[3] Nutbeam D. Health literacy as a public health goal: a challenge for contemporary health education and communication strategies into the 21st century. Health Promot Int 2000;15(3):259-67.

[4] Hamilton LC, Hartter J, Lemcke-Stampone M, Moore DW, Safford TG. Tracking public beliefs about anthropogenic climate change. PLoS One 2015;10(9):e0138208.

[5] Brody JG, Dunagan SC, Morello-Frosch R, Brown P, Patton S, Rudel RA. Reporting individual results for biomonitoring and environmental exposures: lessons learned from environmental communication case studies. Environ Health 2014;13(1):40.

[6] Ramirez-Andreotta MD, Brody JG, Lothrop N, Loh M, Beamer PI, Brown P. Improving environmental health literacy and justice through environmental exposure results communication. Int J Environ Res Public Health 2016;13(7):690.

[7] Brody JG, Brown P, Morello-Frosch RA. Returning chemical exposure results to individuals and communities. Finn S, O'Fallon LR, eds, Environmental health literacy. Cham: Springer; 2019:135-63.

[8] Rohlman D, Donatuto J, Heidt M, Barton M, Campbell L, Anderson KA, et al. A case study describing a community-engaged approach for evaluating polycyclic aromatic hydrocarbon exposure in a native American community. Int J Environ Res Public Health 2019;16(3):327.

[9] National Academies of Sciences E, Medicine. Returning individual research results to participants: guidance for a new research paradigm. Washington, DC: National Academies Press, 2018.

[10] Nelson JW, Scammell MK, Altman RG, Webster TF, Ozonoff DM. A new spin on research translation: the Boston Consensus Conference on Human Biomonitoring. Environ Health Perspect 2009;117(4):495-9.

[11] Dunagan S, Brody J, Morello-Frosch R, Brown P, Goho S, Tovar J, et al. When pollution is personal: Handbook for reporting results to participants in biomonitoring and personal exposure studies. Newton, MA: Silent Spring Institute, 2013:2018-11.

[12] Rohlman D, Kile ML, Irvin VL. Developing a Short Assessment of Environmental Health Literacy (SA-EHL). Int J Environ Res Public Health 2022;19(4):2062.

[13] Irvin VL, Rohlman D, Vaughan A, Amantia R, Berlin C, Kile ML. Development and validation of an environmental health literacy assessment screening tool for domestic well owners: The water environmental literacy level scale (WELLS). Int J Environ Res Public Health 2019;16(5):881.

[14] Gray KM, Triana V, Lindsey M, Richmond B, Hoover AG, Wiesen C. Knowledge and beliefs associated with environmental health literacy: A case study focused on toxic metals contamination of well water. Int J Environ Res Public Health 2021;18(17):9298.

[15] Dixon HM, Bramer LM, Scott RP, Calero L, Holmes D, Gibson EA, et al. Evaluating predictive relationships between wristbands and urine for assessment of personal PAH exposure. Environ Int 2022;163:107226.

[16] Andersson JT, Achten C. Time to say goodbye to the 16 EPA PAHs? Toward an up-to-date use of PACs for environmental purposes. Polycycl Aromat Compd 2015;35(2-4):330-54.

[17] Agency for Toxic Substances and Disease Registry. ATSDR's Substance Priority List Atlanta, GA: ATSDR, 2020. URL: https://www.atsdr.cdc.gov/spl/index.html#2019spl.

[18] Agency for Toxic Substances and Disease Registry. Toxicological profile for polycyclic aromatic hydrocarbons. Atlanta, GA: Division of Toxicology/Toxicology Information Branch, 1995.

[19] Dixon HM, Calero L, Anderson KA, Herbstman J, Rohlman D. Wristband report YouTube: Oregon State University; Columbia University, 2018. URL: https://www.youtube.com/watch?v = 1gVEwf54Z6s.

[20] Gray KM, Lindsey M. Measuring environmental health literacy. In: Finn S, O'Fallon L, eds. Environmental health literacy. Cham: Springer, 2019:19-43.

[21] Porter MF. Snowball: A language for stemming algorithms, 2001. URL: https://snowballstem.org/texts/introduction.html.

[22] Mohammad S, Turney P, eds. Emotions evoked by common words and phrases: Using mechanical turk to create an emotion lexicon. Proceedings of the NAACL HLT 2010 workshop on computational approaches to analysis and generation of emotion in text. Los Angeles, CA, 2010.

[23] Gray KM. From content knowledge to community change: A review of representations of environmental health literacy. Int J Environ Res Public Health 2018;15(3):466.

[24] Dixon JK, Hendrickson KC, Ercolano E, Quackenbush R, Dixon JP. The environmental health engagement profile: What people think and do about environmental health. Public Health Nurs 2009;26(5):460-73.

[25] Lichtveld MY, Covert HH, Sherman M, Shankar A, Wickliffe JK, Alcala CS. Advancing environmental health literacy: Validated scales of general environmental health and environmental media-specific knowledge, attitudes and behaviors Int J Environ Res Public Health 2019;16(21):4157.

[26] Ratnapradipa D, Middleton WK, Wodika AB, Brown SL, Preihs K. What does the public know about environmental health? A qualitative approach to refining an environmental health awareness instrument. J Environ Health 2015;77(8):22-9.

[27] Binder AR, May K, Murphy J, Gross A, Carlsten E. Environmental health literacy as knowing, feeling, and believing: Analyzing linkages between race, ethnicity, and socioeconomic status and willingness to engage in protective behaviors against health threats. Int J Environ Res Public Health 2022;19(5):2701.

[28] Brody JG, Cirillo PM, Boronow KE, Laurie H, Marj P, Susmann HP, et al. Outcomes from returning individual versus only study-wide biomonitoring results in an environmental exposure study using the digital exposure Report-Back Interface (DERBI). Environ Health Perspect 2021;129(11):117005.

[29] Adams C, Brown P, Morello-Frosch R, Brody JG, Rudel R, Zota A, et al. Disentangling the exposure experience: the roles of community context and report-back of environmental exposure data. J Health Soc Behav 2011;52(2):180-96.
[30] Altman RG, Morello-Frosch R, Brody JG, Rudel R, Brown P, Averick M. Pollution comes home and gets personal: women's experience of household chemical exposure. J Health Soc Behav 2008;49(4):417-35.
[31] Morello-Frosch R, Brody JG, Brown P, Altman RG, Rudel RA, Pérez C. Toxic ignorance and right-to-know in biomonitoring results communication: a survey of scientists and study participants. Environ Health 2009;8(1):6.
[32] Perovich LJ, Ohayon JL, Cousins EM, Morello-Frosch R, Brown P, Adamkiewicz G, et al. Reporting to parents on children's exposures to asthma triggers in low-income and public housing, an interview-based case study of ethics, environmental literacy, individual action, and public health benefits. Environ Health 2018;17(1):48.
[33] Garcia-Codina O, Juvinyà-Canal D, Amil-Bujan P, Bertran-Noguer C, González-Mestre MA, Masachs-Fatjo E, et al. Determinants of health literacy in the general population: Results of the Catalan health survey. BMC Public Health 2019;19(1):1122-.
[34] Rohlman D, Frey G, Kile ML, Harper B, Harris S, Motorykin O, et al. Communicating results of a dietary exposure study following consumption of traditionally smoked salmon. Environ Justice 2016;9(3):85-92.
[35] Brown P, Morello-Frosch R, Brody JG, Altman RG, Rudel RA, Senier L, et al. Institutional review board challenges related to community-based participatory research on human exposure to environmental toxins: A case study. Environ Health 2010;9(1):1-12.
[36] Burke K, Calero L, Dixon HM, Barton M, Anderson KA, Herbstman J, et al. Evaluation of Report-Back tools for sharing participant results from passive wristband sampling for polycyclic aromatic hydrocarbons (PAH) [Poster]. Durham, NC: Partnerships for Environmental Public Health 2018 Dec 13-14.

Section two: Acknowledgements

About the editors

I Leslie Rubin, MD, is originally from South Africa where he trained in pediatrics and emigrated to the United States in 1976. He is currently Associate Professor in the Department of Pediatrics at Morehouse School of Medicine, Adjunct Associate Professor, Department of Pediatrics, Emory University School of Medicine, Director of Break the Cycle Program at the Southeast Pediatric Environmental Health Unit at Emory University (PEHSU), President and Founder of Break the Cycle of Health Disparities Inc, and Medical Director of The Rubin Center for Autism and Developmental Pediatrics in Atlanta, Georgia. He has been involved in the health care of children and adults with intellectual and developmental disabilities since 1977. In 1989, he and Allen Crocker published the first textbook on medical care for children and adults with developmental disabilities with the second edition in 2006. Sadly, Allen Crocker passed away in 2011, but, in partnership with Joav Merrick and others published the 3rd edition: "Health care for people with intellectual and developmental disabilities across the lifespan" with Springer in 2016. He currently directs interdisciplinary clinical programs for children with autism, cerebral palsy and other developmental disabilities and consults to a variety of programs including the Emory University Neurodevelopmental Exposure Clinic (ENEC), an interdisciplinary, research-based program looking at the impact of prenatal exposures on child development and behavior in the context of the social and economic disadvantage and health disparities. Among his awards for various activities, he received the Robert E Cooke Lifetime Achievement Award from the AADMD in 2015 and the Autism Achievement Award in 2016 from the Annual Conference and Exposition of Georgia, and the F Edwards Rushton CATCH Award from the American Academy of Pediatric in 2018, and most recently, was named one of 50 Advocate Heroes over the 50 years of Exceptional Parent Magazine. He is actively involved in the American Academy of Pediatrics as the Chair of the Georgia Chapter Environmental Health Committee and District X CATCH Facilitator for the AAP. He was on the US Environmental Protection Agency Board of Scientific Counsellors focusing on Sustainable Healthy

Communities from 2016-2022 and is now on the National Advisory Council for Children and Disasters. He is also the Chair of the National PEHSU Steering Committee and is on the Advisory Councils of HERCULES, the Human Exposome Research Center at Emory University; and on the National START Advisory Committee, based at the University of New Hampshire. In 2004 he founded the Break the Cycle program which addresses children's environmental health disparities by recruiting bright university students to develop creative projects that will Break the Cycle and then publish their papers in international journals and books on public health. To date there have been more than 150 students from the USA, Latin America and Africa. The program received the Children's Environmental Health Excellence Award from the EPA in 2016. Email: lrubi01@emory.edu

Joav Merrick, MD, MMedSci, DMSc, born and educated in Denmark is professor of pediatrics, Division of Pediatrics, Hadassah Hebrew University Medical Center, Mt Scopus Campus, Jerusalem, Israel and Kentucky Children's Hospital, University of Kentucky, Lexington, Kentucky United States and professor of public health at the Center for Healthy Development, School of Public Health, Georgia State University, Atlanta, United States, the former medical director of the Health Services, Division for Intellectual and Developmental Disabilities, Ministry of Social Affairs and Social Services, Jerusalem, the founder and director of the National Institute of Child Health and Human Development in Israel. Numerous publications in the field of pediatrics, child health and human development, rehabilitation, intellectual disability, disability, health, welfare, abuse, advocacy, quality of life and prevention. Received the Peter Sabroe Child Award for outstanding work on behalf of Danish Children in 1985 and the International LEGO-Prize ("The Children's Nobel Prize") for an extraordinary contribution towards improvement in child welfare and well-being in 1987. In 2017 appointed a Kentucky Colonel by the Commonwealth of Kentucky, the highest honor the governor can bestow to a person. Email: jmerrick@zahav.net.il

About the Break the Cycle of Health Disparities Inc

Break the Cycle of Health Disparities Inc. (BCHD) is a private, not-for-profit 501c3, non-governmental organization dedicated to exploring the social, economic and environmental determinants of health in the context of children's health disparities and to use this to promote health equity for all children.

BCHD collaborates with the Southeast PEHSU to produce the annual Break the Cycle of Children's Environmental Health Disparities Program (Break the Cycle). Break the Cycle is a multidisciplinary academic research and training program that focuses on raising awareness of children's environmental health disparities and cultivating future leaders among university students in the fields of medicine, nursing, public health, law, social work, education and other related disciplines.

Each year, Break the Cycle invites students from a diversity of colleges and universities to develop projects that will "break the cycle of children's environmental health disparities". Break the Cycle faculty guides and monitors the progress of the students towards compeltion of their projects. The students present their completed projects at a national conference and their work is published in international journals. Over the past 15 years Break the Cycle has engaged over 150 students from 50 different university departments in 12 states in the USA, as well as students from Latin America, Europe and Africa, that have resulted in the publication of 13 journal supplements. These sets of projects form the basis for this book series.

In 2016, Break the Cycle received a Children's Environmental Health Excellence Award from the US Environmental Protection Agency for the achievements of the program.

BCHD has expanded its areas of interest and practice to Break the Cycle of Autism Disparities, Break the Cycle of Climate Change for Vulnerable Children, Break the Cycle of Environmental Degradation, Break the Cycle of

Children's Mental Health Disparities, and Break the Cycle of Health Disparities for Native Children.

Contact
I Leslie Rubin MD
Associate Professor, Department of Pediatrics,
Morehouse School of Medicine
Adjuct Associate Profesor, Department of Pediatrics,
Emory University School of Medicine
Director, Break the Cycle Program, Southeast Pediatric Environmental Health Specialty Unit, Emory University School of Medicine
President and Founder, Break the Cycle of Health Disparities Inc
Medical Director, The Rubin Center for Autism and
Developmental Pediatrics
750 Hammond Drive, Building 1, Suite 100, Atlanta, GA 30328,
United States
Email: lrubi01@emory.edu
Website: www.breakthecycleprogram.org
Website: www.therubincenterforautism.org

About the Pediatric Environmental Health Specialty Units (PEHSU)

The Pediatric Environmental Health Specialty Units (PEHSU's) are an interconnected system of regional centers located throughout the United States that respond to questions from public health professionals, clinicians, policy makers, and the public about environmental health concerns related to children and reproductive age adults. After fifteen years of programmatic operations, collaborations, and a growing desire to protect the health of children and reproductive age adults from environmental hazards, the PEHSU Program has gained the attention and respect of the pediatric and reproductive environmental medical community and families at risk from exposure to environmental contaminants. The PEHSU programs have a critical role in supporting the mission of the Agency for Toxic Substances and Disease Registry (ATSDR) to prevent or mitigate the adverse human health effects and diminished quality of life that result from exposure to hazardous substances in the environment and the mission of the US Environmental Protection Agency (EPA) to protect human health and the environment. The PEHSUs provide a credible, academic, non-commercial source of health information and clinical expertise regarding environmental toxins and their effects on children and reproductive age adults.

ATSDR and EPA established the PEHSUs to increase the capacity of health care providers to identify and treat environmental-related health conditions, prevent exposure to children and reproductive age adults, and communicate health risks from environmental exposures. The PEHSU Network includes teams of medical specialists (pediatricians, medical toxicologists, obstetricians, nurses, nurse practitioners, occupational and environmental health physicians), public health professionals, researchers, psychologists, and educators to provide consultations, trainings, referrals and clinical services to health care providers, governmental agencies and the general public on pediatric and reproductive environmental health. PEHSUs also engage communities and stakeholders in public outreach projects.

About the Pediatric Environmental Health Specialty Units (PEHSU)

The National PEHSU Network helps individuals and communities to make informed decisions regarding environmental health concerns. Common concerns include lead poisoning, fungus or mold, pesticides, phthalates, air quality and school safety. There have also been national responses generated for hazards from wildfires, hurricanes, oil spills, carbon monoxide, mercury spills, de-icer leaks at airports, and industrial pollution.

While Poison Control Centers respond to acute toxic exposures, the PEHSU Network has expertise in long term, chronic low dose exposures, group exposures, and the development and dissemination of public messages. The PEHSU Network partners closely with local, state, and federal agencies and non-profit professional organizations in carrying out this work.

The PEHSUs collaborate with ATSDR and EPA to develop fact sheets targeting clinicians and the public on issues associated with flooding, hurricanes, wildfires, oil spills, formaldehyde, carbon monoxide poisoning, arsenic in foods, medical management of lead exposure, phthalates and bisphenol A, melamine, and other issues. They edit academic textbooks, publish manuscripts, and conduct outreach and educational programs to enhance pediatric and reproductive environmental health literacy.

The PEHSU's provide information online (website: www.pehsu.net) with a variety of materials to educate professionals and the general public in reproductive and children's environmental health through conferences, presentations and social media. PEHSU members serve on national boards and committees to advance collaborative activities and community expertise in environmental health. The PEHSUs train and mentor medical, toxicology, nursing, and other graduate students and provide hands-on opportunities in pediatric environmental medicine and reproductive epidemiology. The PEHSUs have advised first responders, parents, health officials, and school administrators on how to assess and mitigate environmental emergencies and address health-related findings. They have also provided training to establish PEHSUs in Chile, Argentina, Canada, Mexico, Vietnam, and Israel.

The PEHSUs serve to translate research findings into clinical and public health practice. PEHSU faculty are prepared to recognize, treat, and prevent toxic environmental exposures in children and communicate risk, treatment, and prevention strategies in a meaningful and culturally appropriate way.

Southeast PEHSU

The Southeast PEHSU, within the National PEHSU network, serves the southeastern United States and includes Alabama, North Carolina, South Carolina, Florida, Georgia, Kentucky, Mississippi and Tennessee. The Southeast PEHSU is based in the Nell Hodgson Woodruff School of Nursing at Emory University in Atlanta, GA and works closely with Region 4 of the US Environmental Protection Agency (EPA) and the Agency for Toxic Substances and Disease Registry (ATSDR) at the Centers for Disease Control and Prevention (CDC). The team includes Abby Mutic, PhD, MSN, CNM (Assistant Professor and Certified Nurse Midwife), Leslie Rubin, MD (Developmental Pediatrician), Melissa Gittinger, DO (Medical Toxicologist), Rebecca Philipsborn, MD, MPA (Pediatrician), Victoria Green, MD, JD, MBA (Obstetrician Gynecologist), Henry Falk, MD MPH (Formerly Director of ATSDR), Nathan Mutic, MS, MAT, MEd (Educator and Program Administrator), and Wayne Garfinkel, BSCE (formerly of Region 4 EPA). In addition, Benjamin Gitterman, MD (Pediatrician) works with the Southeast PEHSU on the Break the Cycle program.

Contact Southeast PEHSU
Abby Mutic, PhD, MSN, CNM
Director, Southeast Pediatric Environmental Health Specialty Unit
Nell Hodgson Woodruff School of Nursing, Emory University
1520 Clifton Road, Atlanta, GA 30322, United States.
Toll free tel: (877) 33 PEHSU or (877) 337-3478
Tel: (404) 727-7980
E-mail: sepehsu@emory.edu
Website: https://www.nursing.emory.edu/pages/southeastern-pediatric-environmental-health-specialty-unit

About the National Institute of Child Health and Human Development in Israel

The National Institute of Child Health and Human Development (NICHD) in Israel was established in 1998 as a virtual institute under the auspices of the Medical Director, Ministry of Social Affairs and Social Services in order to function as the research arm for the Office of the Medical Director. In 1998 the National Council for Child Health and Pediatrics, Ministry of Health and in 1999 the Director General and Deputy Director General of the Ministry of Health endorsed the establishment of the NICHD.

Mission

The mission of a National Institute for Child Health and Human Development in Israel is to provide an academic focal point for the scholarly interdisciplinary study of child life, health, public health, welfare, disability, rehabilitation, intellectual disability and related aspects of human development. This mission includes research, teaching, clinical work, information and public service activities in the field of child health and human development.

Service and academic activities

Over the years many activities became focused in the south of Israel due to collaboration with various professionals at the Faculty of Health Sciences (FOHS) at the Ben Gurion University of the Negev (BGU). Since 2000 an affiliation with the Zusman Child Development Center at the Pediatric Division of Soroka University Medical Center has resulted in collaboration around the establishment of the Down Syndrome Clinic at that center. In 2002 a full course on "Disability" was established at the Recanati School for Allied Professions in the Community, FOHS, BGU and in 2005 collaboration was started with the Primary Care Unit of the faculty and disability became part of the master of public health course on "Children and society". In the academic year 2005-2006 a one semester course on "Aging with disability" was started as part of the master of science program in gerontology in our collaboration with the Center for Multidisciplinary Research in Aging. In 2010 collaborations with the Division of Pediatrics, Hadassah Hebrew University Medical Center, Jerusalem, Israel around the National Down Syndrome Center and teaching students and residents about intellectual and developmental disabilities as part of their training at this campus.

Research activities

The affiliated staff have over the years published work from projects and research activities in this national and international collaboration. In the year 2000 the International Journal of Adolescent Medicine and Health and in 2005 the International Journal on Disability and Human Development of De Gruyter Publishing House (Berlin and New York) were affiliated with the National Institute of Child Health and Human Development. From 2008 also the International Journal of Child Health and Human Development (Nova Science, New York), the International Journal of Child and Adolescent Health (Nova Science) and the Journal of Pain Management (Nova Science) affiliated and from 2009 the International Public Health Journal (Nova Science) and Journal of Alternative Medicine Research (Nova Science). All peer-reviewed international journals.

National collaborations

Nationally the NICHD works in collaboration with the Faculty of Health Sciences, Ben Gurion University of the Negev; Department of Physical Therapy, Sackler School of Medicine, Tel Aviv University; Autism Center, Assaf HaRofeh Medical Center; National Rett and PKU Centers at Chaim Sheba Medical Center, Tel HaShomer; Department of Physiotherapy, Haifa University; Department of Education, Bar Ilan University, Ramat Gan, Faculty of Social Sciences and Health Sciences; College of Judea and Samaria in Ariel and in 2011 affiliation with Center for Pediatric Chronic Diseases and National Center for Down Syndrome, Department of Pediatrics, Hadassah Hebrew University Medical Center, Mount Scopus Campus, Jerusalem.

International collaborations

Internationally with the Department of Disability and Human Development, College of Applied Health Sciences, University of Illinois at Chicago; Strong Center for Developmental Disabilities, Golisano Children's Hospital at Strong, University of Rochester School of Medicine and Dentistry, New York; Centre on Intellectual Disabilities, University of Albany, New York; Centre for Chronic Disease Prevention and Control, Health Canada, Ottawa; Chandler Medical Center and Children's Hospital, Kentucky Children's Hospital, Section of Adolescent Medicine, University of Kentucky, Lexington; Chronic Disease Prevention and Control Research Center, Baylor College of Medicine, Houston, Texas; Division of Neuroscience, Department of Psychiatry, Columbia University, New York; Institute for the Study of Disadvantage and Disability, Atlanta; Center for Autism and Related Disorders, Department Psychiatry, Children's Hospital Boston, Boston; Department of Pediatric and Adolescent Medicine, Western Michigan University Homer Stryker MD School of Medicine, Kalamazoo, Michigan, United States; Department of Paediatrics, Child Health and Adolescent Medicine, Children's Hospital at Westmead, Westmead, Australia; International Centre for the Study of Occupational and Mental Health, Düsseldorf, Germany; Centre for Advanced Studies in Nursing, Department of General Practice and Primary Care, University of Aberdeen, Aberdeen, United Kingdom; Quality of Life Research Center, Copenhagen, Denmark; Nordic School of Public Health, Gottenburg, Sweden, Scandinavian Institute of Quality of Working Life, Oslo, Norway; The Department of Applied Social Sciences (APSS) of The Hong Kong Polytechnic University Hong Kong.

Targets

Our focus is on research, international collaborations, clinical work, teaching and policy in health, disability and human development and to establish the

NICHD as a permanent institute in Israel in order to conduct model research and provide policy aspects in the field of interest.

Contact
Professor Joav Merrick, MD, MMedSci, DMSc
Director, National Institute of Child Health and Human Development, Jerusalem, Israel. E-mail: jmerrick@zahav.net.il

Section three: Index

Index

A

access to quality healthcare, 4, 18
adolescents, 9, 13, 38, 45, 48, 49, 50, 76, 120
African American, 8, 12, 15, 25, 26, 28, 31, 34, 76, 82, 89, 94
attention deficit hyperactivity disorder (ADHD), 5, 97, 134
autism spectrum disorders (ASD), 13, 38, 40, 43, 44, 47, 48

B

behavior problems, 5
Black, 8, 14, 28, 31, 52, 63, 67, 70, 76, 84, 89, 90, 94, 95, 125, 151
blood, 5, 12, 14, 15, 20, 25, 29, 30, 31, 32, 36, 51, 52, 54, 55, 59, 61, 62, 63, 64, 65, 66, 67, 68, 69, 70, 72, 74, 75, 76, 77, 78, 82, 83, 84, 86, 87, 89, 92, 93, 94, 95, 96, 97, 98, 99, 105, 114, 151
Bolivia, 40
Brazil, 40
Break the Cycle (BTC), v, vi, 3, 4, 9, 10, 11, 12, 13, 14, 18, 19, 22, 23, 25, 26, 28, 29, 30, 31, 32, 33, 34, 37, 39, 40, 41, 42, 44, 45, 46, 47, 48, 49, 74, 106, 113, 114, 131, 132, 152, 154, 165, 167, 168, 171

C

Caribbean, 38, 39, 49
Centers for Disease Control and Prevention (CDC), 9, 21, 22, 47, 73, 74, 83, 92, 97, 113, 121, 171
child health, vi, 4, 8, 17, 21, 36, 39, 49, 77, 104, 112, 117, 118, 119, 121, 124, 132, 133, 166, 173, 174, 175, 176
childhood, 14, 17, 20, 21, 32, 36, 40, 51, 52, 53, 73, 74, 75, 76, 78, 85, 97, 106, 107, 114, 117, 120, 130, 140
children, 3, 4, 5, 6, 7, 8, 9, 10, 11, 12, 13, 14, 15, 16, 17, 18, 19, 20, 21, 25, 29, 30, 31, 32, 36, 38, 39, 40, 42, 43, 44, 45, 47, 48, 49, 50, 51, 52, 53, 54, 55, 56, 57, 58, 59, 60, 62, 63, 64, 65, 66, 67, 68, 69, 70, 71, 72, 73, 74, 75, 76, 77, 78, 81, 82, 83, 84, 85, 86, 95, 96, 98, 99, 101, 102, 103, 105, 106, 107, 111, 114, 118, 122, 123, 124, 125, 130, 132, 133, 134, 135, 137, 139, 140, 151, 161, 165, 166, 167, 169, 170, 174, 175
Chile, 13, 37, 39, 40, 41, 42, 43, 45, 47, 49, 50, 170
community factors, 63, 67
community water service, 13, 26, 28, 29, 30, 32, 33, 34, 69, 70, 84
community water service access, 28

D

dust, 12, 15, 25, 48, 65, 72, 75, 82, 86, 87, 88, 89, 92, 93, 96, 103, 108

E

environmental factors, 4, 5, 8, 9, 10, 14, 19, 31, 40, 51, 52, 94, 103, 112
environmental health disparities, 3, 7, 8, 9, 11, 12, 19, 21, 49, 74, 85, 86, 104, 106, 130, 132, 139, 152, 166, 167
environmental health literacy (EHL), vi, 14, 17, 18, 106, 111, 112, 115, 137, 138, 139, 142, 143, 144, 146, 147, 149, 150, 151, 152, 158, 159, 160, 170
environmental pediatrics, 42
exclusion criteria, 55

extraterritorial jurisdictions (ETJs), 26, 27, 28, 29, 30, 33
extremely low gestational age newborn (ELGAN), 17, 117, 118, 119, 122, 123, 124, 125, 130, 131, 132, 133, 134

G

Guatemala, 40

H

health disparities, vi, 3, 4, 9, 10, 18, 19, 22, 26, 40, 47, 74, 75, 103, 106, 113, 114, 130, 165, 167, 168
Hispanic, 8, 14, 31, 52, 63, 67, 83, 89, 90, 125, 139, 140, 142, 145, 151, 152
Hispanic American children, 8

I

inclusion criteria, 55, 56
indoor environmental risk factors, 13, 38, 41, 43
indoor risk factors, 40
institutional factors, 66
interpersonal factors, 64
intrapersonal factors, 60, 63

L

Latin America, v, 9, 11, 13, 37, 38, 39, 40, 41, 46, 47, 49, 166, 167
Latin American communities, v, 13, 37
lead (Pb), v, 5, 6, 12, 14, 15, 16, 20, 25, 29, 30, 31, 32, 33, 34, 36, 48, 51, 52, 53, 54, 55, 56, 58, 59, 60, 61, 62, 63, 64, 65, 66, 67, 68, 69, 70, 71, 72, 73, 74, 75, 76, 77, 78, 79, 81, 82, 83, 84, 85, 86, 87, 88, 89, 92, 93, 94, 95, 96, 97, 98, 99, 102, 103,105, 106, 107, 108, 109, 110, 112, 114, 153, 170
lead exposure, v, 6, 14, 15, 16, 36, 51, 52, 54, 74, 76, 77, 78, 81, 82, 83, 84, 85, 87, 88, 89, 97, 98, 102, 103, 106, 107, 109, 110, 114, 170
lead poisoning, 52, 54, 75, 76, 77, 97, 105, 106, 107, 114, 170

M

maternal disorders during pregnancy, vi, 17, 117
maternal education, vi, 17, 117, 118, 119, 122, 123, 124, 125, 130, 131, 132, 135, 142, 143, 144, 146, 150
Mexico, 40, 63, 170

N

national laws, 53
Native American, 8, 12, 15, 25, 82, 94, 95, 96, 125

O

obesity prevention, 40

P

Paraguay, 37, 40
Pediatric Environmental Health Center (PEHC), vi, 16, 101, 102, 105, 106, 107, 110, 112
perfluoroalkyl substances (PFAS), 16, 102, 105, 108, 111, 151
policies, 14, 51, 52, 53, 68, 70, 71
pollution and respiratory symptoms, 40
polycyclic aromatic hydrocarbon exposure, vi, 17, 137, 159
positive child health index (PCHI), 17, 117, 118, 119, 121, 122, 123, 124, 129, 130, 132
poverty, 4, 5, 6, 8, 9, 18, 21, 39, 64, 67, 70, 73, 99, 103, 104
pregnancy vulnerability, 130
private well water, 15, 30, 31, 33, 36, 69, 76, 82, 84, 85, 95, 98, 99

private wells, v, 15, 27, 29, 31, 33, 36, 69, 81, 84, 86, 95, 96
Puerto Rico, 40

R

race/ethnicity, 8, 35, 60, 63, 64, 67, 70, 89, 90, 94, 96, 99, 125, 142, 144, 145, 151, 160
regulations, 26, 53, 66, 97
respiratory diseases, 13, 38, 41, 43, 49, 103
risk factors, 14, 41, 42, 43, 49, 51, 52, 53, 55, 57, 61, 62, 73, 78, 131

S

Safe Drinking Water Act, 15, 70, 81, 83, 84, 97
social determinants of health (SDOH), 13, 38, 40, 41, 102, 105, 107, 114, 118, 130
social-ecological model (SEM), 14, 32, 51, 53, 56, 60, 63, 64, 66, 70, 71, 72, 73

U

underserved communities, 13, 37, 39, 40, 42, 45
United States (US), 8, 9, 11, 14, 15, 20, 31, 35, 36, 51, 52, 54, 58, 63, 64, 71, 73, 74, 75, 76, 77, 78, 79, 82, 83, 84, 95, 96, 97, 98, 113, 165, 167, 169, 171

W

water, v, 5, 6, 12, 14, 15, 25, 26, 27, 28, 29, 30, 31, 32, 33, 34, 35, 36, 38, 52, 56, 63, 68, 69, 70, 72, 76, 78, 81, 83, 84, 85, 86, 87, 88, 89, 90, 91, 92, 93, 94, 95, 96, 97, 98, 99, 103, 105, 108, 159
water quality, 33, 84, 98, 105
White children, 8, 63